ADVANCING THE FEDERAL RESEARCH AGENDA ON
VIOLENCE AGAINST WOMEN

Steering Committee for the Workshop on Issues in
Research on Violence Against Women

Candace Kruttschnitt, Brenda L. McLaughlin, and Carol V. Petrie, editors

Committee on Law and Justice

Division of Behavioral and Social Sciences and Education

NATIONAL RESEARCH COUNCIL
OF THE NATIONAL ACADEMIES

THE NATIONAL ACADEMIES PRESS
Washington, D.C.
www.nap.edu

THE NATIONAL ACADEMIES PRESS 500 Fifth Street, NW Washington, DC 20001

NOTICE: The project that is the subject of this report was approved by the Governing Board of the National Research Council, whose members are drawn from the councils of the National Academy of Sciences, the National Academy of Engineering, and the Institute of Medicine. The members of the committee responsible for the report were chosen for their special competences and with regard for appropriate balance.

This study was supported by the National Academy of Sciences and Grant No. 2000-IJ-CX-0014 from the National Institute of Justice, Office of Justice Programs, U.S. Department of Justice. Any opinions, findings, conclusions, or recommendations expressed in this publication are those of the author(s) and do not necessarily reflect the views of the organizations or agencies that provided support for the project.

Library of Congress Cataloging-in-Publication Data

Advancing the federal research agenda on violence against women / Steering Committee for the Workshop on Issues in Research on Violence Against Women ; Candace Kruttschnitt, Brenda L. McLaughlin, and Carol V. Petrie, editors ; Committee on Law and Justice, Division of Behavioral and Social Sciences and Education, National Research Council of the National Academies.
    p. cm.
Based on a workshop convened by the National Research Council in January 2002.
Includes bibliographical references.
  ISBN 0-309-09109-8 (pbk.) — ISBN 0-309-52838-0 (pdf)
  1. Women—Crimes against—United States—Congresses. 2. Women—Crimes against—Research—United States—Congresses. 3. Women—Violence against—United States—Congresses. 4. Women—Violence against—Research—United States—Congresses. I. Kruttschnitt, Candace. II. McLaughlin, Brenda L. III. Petrie, Carol. IV. National Research Council (U.S.). Steering Committee for the Workshop on Issues in Research on Violence Against Women. V. National Research Council (U.S.). Committee on Law and Justice.
  HV6250.4.W65A38 2004
  362.88'082'0973—dc22

2003026717

Additional copies of this report are available from the National Academies Press, 500 Fifth Street, N.W., Lockbox 285, Washington, DC 20055; (800) 624-6242 or (202) 334-3313 (in the Washington metropolitan area); Internet, http://www.nap.edu.

Printed in the United States of America

Suggested citation: National Research Council. (2004). *Advancing the Federal Research Agenda on Violence Against Women*. Steering Committee for the Workshop on Issues in Research on Violence Against Women, Candace Kruttschnitt, Brenda L. McLaughlin, and Carol V. Petrie, editors. Committee on Law and Justice, Division of Behavioral and Social Sciences and Education. Washington, DC: The National Academies Press.

THE NATIONAL ACADEMIES
Advisers to the Nation on Science, Engineering, and Medicine

The **National Academy of Sciences** is a private, nonprofit, self-perpetuating society of distinguished scholars engaged in scientific and engineering research, dedicated to the furtherance of science and technology and to their use for the general welfare. Upon the authority of the charter granted to it by the Congress in 1863, the Academy has a mandate that requires it to advise the federal government on scientific and technical matters. Dr. Bruce M. Alberts is president of the National Academy of Sciences.

The **National Academy of Engineering** was established in 1964, under the charter of the National Academy of Sciences, as a parallel organization of outstanding engineers. It is autonomous in its administration and in the selection of its members, sharing with the National Academy of Sciences the responsibility for advising the federal government. The National Academy of Engineering also sponsors engineering programs aimed at meeting national needs, encourages education and research, and recognizes the superior achievements of engineers. Dr. Wm. A. Wulf is president of the National Academy of Engineering.

The **Institute of Medicine** was established in 1970 by the National Academy of Sciences to secure the services of eminent members of appropriate professions in the examination of policy matters pertaining to the health of the public. The Institute acts under the responsibility given to the National Academy of Sciences by its congressional charter to be an adviser to the federal government and, upon its own initiative, to identify issues of medical care, research, and education. Dr. Harvey V. Fineberg is president of the Institute of Medicine.

The **National Research Council** was organized by the National Academy of Sciences in 1916 to associate the broad community of science and technology with the Academy's purposes of furthering knowledge and advising the federal government. Functioning in accordance with general policies determined by the Academy, the Council has become the principal operating agency of both the National Academy of Sciences and the National Academy of Engineering in providing services to the government, the public, and the scientific and engineering communities. The Council is administered jointly by both Academies and the Institute of Medicine. Dr. Bruce M. Alberts and Dr. Wm. A. Wulf are chair and vice chair, respectively, of the National Research Council.

www.national-academies.org

Carol Petrie, *Study Director*
Brenda McLaughlin, *Research Associate*
Ralph Patterson, *Senior Project Assistant*

Preface

K nowledge from research on the violent victimization of women has advanced significantly during the past decade. As a result of improved survey research in the fields of criminal justice and public health, we now have a better grasp of the scope and nature of violence against women, especially intimate-partner violence and sexual assault. Much remains to be done, however, especially to increase our knowledge of the causes and consequences of serious assaults, including sexual assaults, and homicides against women. The nation now spends hundreds of millions of dollars to improve the safety of women, especially at home, and yet more than half of all female homicide victims are killed by an intimate partner, other family member, or acquaintance. Although, as with homicide in general, the rates of domestic homicide for women have decreased, they have declined at a slower rate than those for men. In addition, the violent victimization of women by strangers and in other settings and circumstances has been largely neglected in the research literature.

This report expands on the work of an earlier National Research Council (NRC) panel whose report, *Understanding Violence Against Women*, was published in 1996. While some of the research recommended in that report has been funded and carried out, important gaps remain. For example, prevalence and incidence data are still inadequate to measure trends or to reveal whether the interventions being designed are in fact working to improve the overall safety of women in society. It is hoped that the recommendations in the present report will begin to improve this situation.

This report is based on the presentations and deliberations of a workshop convened by the NRC in January 2002 to develop a detailed research agenda on violence against women. The chapters in the report draw on the eight papers commissioned for the workshop, on the comments made by a panel of distinguished commentators, and on the discussion by workshop participants. Many people made generous contributions to the workshop's success. We thank the authors of the papers presented: Laura Dugan and Robert Apel, University of Maryland; Jacquelyn Campbell and Jennifer Manganello, Johns Hopkins University; Sandra Martin and Beth Moracco, University of North Carolina; Juanjo Medina, University of Manchester; Deanna Wilkinson and Susan Hamerschlag, Temple University; Kirk Williams and Elizabeth Conniff, University of California, Riverside; Christopher Maxwell and Lori Post, Michigan State University; Amy Holtzworth-Munroe and Jeffrey Meehan, Indiana University, Bloomington; and Daniel Saunders and Richard Hamill, University of Michigan. We also thank the scholars who prepared comments on each of the papers: Ann Coker, University of South Carolina; Colin Loftin, University at Albany; Ross MacMillan, University of Minnesota; Michael Benson, University of Cincinnati; Robert F. Meier, University of Nebraska; Greg Pogarsky, University at Albany; Alissa Worden, University at Albany; John Firman, International Association of Chiefs of Police; Julie Horney, University at Albany; and Marty Friday, Women's Center and Shelter of Greater Pittsburgh. We thank as well the scholars who presented on topics not covered by the papers: David Ford, Indiana University; Adele Harrell, Urban Institute; Patricia Munhall, University of South Carolina; Beth Richie, University of Illinois, Chicago; Carolyn Rebecca Block, Illinois Criminal Justice Information Authority; Myrna Dawson, University of Western Ontario; and Bill McCarthy, University of California, Davis.

We also thank Kirsten Sampson Snyder, Reports Officer, Rona Briere, editor, and Yvonne Wise for managing the production process.

This report has been reviewed in draft form by individuals chosen for their diverse perspectives and technical expertise, in accordance with procedures approved by the NRC's Report Review Committee. The purpose of this independent review is to provide candid and critical comments that will assist the institution in making its published report as sound as possible and to ensure that the report meets institutional standards for objectivity, evidence, and responsiveness to the study charge. The review comments and draft manuscript remain confidential to protect the integrity of the deliberative process. We wish to thank the following individuals for their review of this report: Rosemary Gartner, Centre of Criminology, University of Toronto; Karen Heimer, Department of Sociology, University of Iowa; Julie Horney, School of Criminal Justice, University at Albany, State University of New York; Catherine Stayton, Department of

Health and Nutrition Sciences, Brooklyn College, City University of New York; and Ralph Brecken Taylor, Department of Criminal Justice, Temple University.

Although the reviewers listed above provided many constructive comments and suggestions, they were not asked to endorse the report's conclusions or recommendations, nor did they see the final draft of the report before its release. The review of this report was overseen by Richard B. Rosenfeld, Department of Criminology and Criminal Justice, University of Missouri-St. Louis. Appointed by the NRC, he was responsible for making certain that an independent examination of this report was carried out in accordance with institutional procedures and that all review comments were carefully considered. Responsibility for the final content of this report rests entirely with the authoring committee and the institution.

Candace Kruttschnitt
Chair

Contents

xi

Executive Summary

Violence against women is a major social problem in the United States, as well as throughout the world. Each year in this country, 300,000 women are forcibly raped, more than 4 million suffer an aggravated or simple assault, and women account for one-fifth of all homicide victims. Moreover, while homicide rates declined during the 1990s for both men and women, the decline in intimate-partner homicides occurred much later in the decade for women than it did for men and was greater for male than for female victims.

In recognition of these continuing problems, in 2000 Congress asked the National Research Council to develop a detailed research agenda on violence against women. To address this mandate, the National Academies appointed a steering committee of four distinguished scholars to develop a workshop that would review research on violence against women, focusing particularly, but not exclusively, on studies completed between 1995 and 2000. The workshop deliberations and the conclusions and recommendations subsequently developed by the steering committee are detailed in this final report.

RESEARCH FOCUS

Because the majority of extant research on violence against women addresses intimate-partner violence, much of this report has a similar focus. The committee notes, however, that two-thirds of homicides against women take place outside of this context, and that violence against women is perpetrated by strangers and acquaintances as well as by domestic part-

1

ners. Moreover, studies of the prevalence of intimate-partner violence show that women themselves commit these acts and not solely for defensive purposes, although at a rate and level of severity far lower than is the case for men.

Most research on violence against women has been conducted in isolation from the larger body of work on violence in general (including research such as that on violence by men, on violence by adolescents, and on criminal careers). This intellectual separation of research on violence against women stems from the premise that distinctive features of the social and political context of violence against women, particularly the context of intimate relationships, sets it apart from other forms of violence. The committee agrees that, as with medical research, a specialized focus on women's victimization and offending behavior is important to ensure that the distinctive correlates and contexts of these phenomena and their aftermath are addressed and receive appropriate funding and attention. However, we urge an end to the almost total separation that has characterized the field.

Since there is still much to be learned about the etiology of violent behavior, the committee questions whether the general origins and behavioral patterns of the various forms of violence are different enough to warrant the degree of separation that has occurred. In fact, recent evidence from longitudinal studies suggests the opposite. The committee believes that research can be focused on a specific issue such as violence against women, but still be firmly grounded in the larger literature on violence generally. **At this point in its development, some level of integration of research on violence against and by women with the larger literature on crime and violence would enrich the former research intellectually, increase the amount of attention it receives, extend the lessons that can be learned about violence against women, and provide a sounder basis for prevention and deterrence strategies.** In addition, findings from research on violence against women could in turn be used to inform research on other types of violence. **The committee also finds that the research agenda of the federal government on violence against women would benefit from its integration with efforts to determine the causes, consequences, prevention, treatment, and deterrence of violence more broadly. Moreover, we believe that the government's research agenda should encompass forms of violent victimization of women other than intimate-partner violence.**

PREVALENCE

Although existing national surveys have provided vital information on the nature and scope of the violent victimization of women over the past 10 years, the information on prevalence and incidence (rates of new cases) is inadequate. Current prevalence information has been derived from methodologically disparate survey data. Survey research has been instrumental in setting some parameters for the scope of two types of violence—intimate-partner violence and sexual assault. Nevertheless, survey research has been less successful in providing reliable estimates of the prevalence and incidence of such violence, as well as information about the context in which it occurs, its developmental patterns over time, and the ways in which women's victimization experiences may be linked to women's offending behaviors. Only a handful of current surveys that collect self-report victimization information from women are continuous; most have varied in the sampling frames and survey instruments used, and most were designed with other purposes in mind.

If trends are to be estimated and the general effectiveness of interventions assessed, prevalence data must be improved. The committee recommends a more coordinated research strategy to help remedy this problem. The committee also recommends that an effort be made to investigate how to link existing datasets and how to link information from these datasets with findings from clinical research. This effort should include creating a framework for developing standard definitions to overcome the lack of conceptual and operational clarity, comparable samples, and interview protocols.

The steering committee believes that a program of research to assess what can be learned from extant data sources might provide important information on prevalence and on how best to proceed to develop more accurate datasets—especially whether a new and continuous national survey is needed. This assessment might also show whether linking existing data can provide more information on the risks of, responses to, and consequences of violence against women and the impacts of interventions.

CAUSES OF VIOLENCE AGAINST WOMEN

A growing body of empirical evidence reveals that perpetrators of violence against women commonly have histories of violence and conduct problems outside of intimate relationships; the same is also true for women who perpetrate violent behavior. However, there is no longitudinal sample of the U.S. population currently examining causes of violence against or by women.

The steering committee agrees with workshop presenters and attendees that information from longitudinal studies of U.S. populations is needed to examine the causes and consequences of violence against and by women. Studies that address risk factors for women should have female respondents, but longitudinal population-based studies that include both men and women also are critical. The latter studies are essential for designing and evaluating the effects of primary prevention strategies and for determining causes, especially the extent to which childhood precursors of violent delinquency and adult crime are at the root of partner violence or other forms of violence against women. The design of data collection systems in such studies should follow from the research questions of interest and should advance general knowledge of violent behavior and its consequences. **The committee recognizes that new funding would be needed for longitudinal studies on violence against women, and believes that the National Institutes of Health and the National Institute of Justice should collaborate on the design and implementation of such studies. The committee recommends that work be initiated to examine the feasibility and cost-effectiveness of successfully conducting longitudinal studies on violence against and by women.**

EVENT-BASED STUDIES

Recent studies on interpersonal violence among strangers illustrate the confluence of several contextual factors—including motivation, perceptions of risk and opportunity, and social control attributes of the setting—that shapes the decision to perpetrate a violent event, as well as its outcome. To understand the catalyst for a violent event among intimates, researchers must examine male–female relationships, perceived imbalances in power, control dynamics, identity threats, relationship problems, and communication patterns. Such event-based research would complement studies of the individual propensities of offenders, focusing instead on the occurrence of violence by identifying the specific conditions that channel individual motivation and predispositions into violent actions, as well as the responses of the justice and health care systems and the community. **The committee therefore recommends more research addressing the situational contexts and dynamic interactions that lead to violence against women. Special attention should be given to research on the processes underlying victim selection, location selection, and victim–offender interaction patterns.**

SOCIAL ECOLOGICAL STUDIES

An emerging body of research provides evidence for community effects on violence and social problems in cases in which gender is an issue. Within the past several years, a number of studies have shown that rates of violence against women vary across such social areas as census tracts and neighborhoods, and that the geographic distribution of violent victimization of women overlaps to a large degree with that of male victimization. These findings are perhaps easier to understand once we confront the fact that most violence against both men and women is perpetrated by men.

Social and Spatial Epidemiology of Violence

The committee believes that current prevalence estimates for acts of stranger-perpetrated violence such as robbery, assault, and rape may be conservative for the neighborhoods in which poor women of color live, and that this exposure to violence by strangers may contribute to factors that characterize violent offending by women. Even intimate-partner violence appears to be susceptible to neighborhood effects. **The committee recommends research to estimate the extent of variation in violence against women among census tracts or small neighborhoods, police precincts or districts, or other theoretically meaningful social area aggregations. Research should also be aimed at determining which features of area composition influence rates and types of violence against women.** Understanding the social structural, social organizational, and social control capacities of neighborhoods is critical to explaining differences in rates of violence against women. This research should compare data across gender in order to determine any differences between male victimization and violence against women.

Distribution of Services

Availability of services has been linked to variation in rates of intimate-partner homicides against women. **The committee recommends that research examine whether access to local services can affect localized rates of intimate-partner violence, and consider implications for planning and locating preventive services.** Research should examine, for example, the relationship between violence "hot spots" and service locations to assess distances that pose barriers to the prevention or deterrence of intimate-partner violence. Research on the locations of other services, including counseling centers and medical services, should examine this relationship as well.

Social Area Effects on Sanctions and Services

Social ecological factors may affect not only rates of violence, but also the efficacy of legal sanctions and social interventions. **The committee recommends that research examine the covariation of individual and social area factors with the responses of both victims and offenders to legal sanctions and social interventions directed at violence against**

women. Whether area effects are mediators or moderators of legal sanctions or social interventions is a question of theoretical and practical importance in the prevention of violence against women.

Data Needs

To create a data infrastructure that can incorporate social ecological factors, modifications will be needed in the sampling strategies used in survey research and epidemiological studies. **Stratified sampling designs in survey and epidemiological research should include samples of social areas as well as of individuals within areas. The selection of social areas, along with the types of data collected, should reflect theoretical questions.** For example, studies of informal social control should include survey data from individuals within the salient areas who can report on social organization and dynamic processes of social control.

PREVENTION AND TREATMENT

The committee notes that the evaluation literature on the effects of prevention and treatment strategies is particularly weak. As a previous National Research Council committee found, the design of prevention and control strategies—programs and services available to victims and offenders that aim to decrease the number of new cases of assault or abusive behavior, reduce the risk of death or disability from violence, and extend life after a violent event—frequently is driven by ideology and stakeholder interests rather than by plausible theories and scientific evidence of causes. Many evaluations were initiated only after programs had been fully implemented in the field. The research on outcomes of treatment—programs and services aimed at changing the behavior of violent offenders— has only begun to emerge, and is in general of poor quality. Evaluations are rarely experimental and thus are unable to rule out nontreatment effects, or they rely on official records that underestimate rates of violence. In most cases, follow-up periods for measuring reoffending or other long-term outcomes are of insufficient length. Another problem is that treatment outcomes have not been uniformly identified, conceptualized, or operationalized.

Instead of using post hoc evaluation designs, it may be more helpful to use standard research and development methods, that is, to design a program around established theory and then test its effects. Where experimental designs are not possible or feasible, such as in evaluating multidimensional, community-wide interventions, other methods, such as the use of propensity scores or econometric models, may yield valid and reliable results. Such rigorous evaluations are lacking for most prevention and treatment approaches. This lack is due primarily to the low level of funding provided for program evaluation in this area; current funding levels make experimental or prospective designs in particular unsupportable.

The committee recommends that Congress provide adequate funds to support rigorous research designs and long-term evaluations of prevention and treatment programs in order to improve chances of effecting long-term reductions in the violent victimization of women. Because of inherent conflicts of interest (no program wants to be found ineffective), funds for program evaluation must be independent from the control of program sponsors so that the ability to evaluate interventions will not be constrained by legislative or other requirements placed on programs or by political considerations. **The steering committee recommends that, because of their individual histories in conducting research and demonstration work on these issues, the National Institutes of Health and the National Institute of Justice collaborate to develop an integrated program of rigorous evaluations of prevention, intervention, treatment, and control strategies.**

DETERRENCE

Most of the research on deterrence—the use of sanctions to prevent offenders from using violence—has focused on specific deterrence aimed at those who have already offended, with the goal of reducing repeat intimate-partner violence. This research shows that legal sanctions do have deterrent effects, although modest in magnitude, but that these effects vary by characteristics of perpetrators, their relationship with their partners, their stake in social conformity, and factors influencing the decision to impose sanctions. Recent research also indicates that certain legal reforms or changes in sanctions for intimate-partner violence, such as imposing more-certain or in some instances more-severe sanctions or reducing opportunities to assault women physically or sexually, increase general deterrence (defined as the impact of legal sanctions on the larger population, that is, those who have neither violated the law nor been punished).

While research shows that the collective actions of the criminal justice system exert a substantial deterrent effect on crime, this fact is of limited value in formulating policy for specific crime problems. **The committee recommends that future research on deterring violence against women be folded into broader efforts to study the decision making of potential perpetrators and the deterrence of criminal behavior generally.** This is a particularly important point given the scope and cost of program efforts aimed at deterring and preventing violence against women. The committee believes that research in the following areas is critical to improving the ability to deter violence against women.

The Long-Term Effects of Sanctioning Policies. If the principal deterrent effect of formal sanctions for violence against women (or other crimes) derives from fear of social stigma, the extent to which such penalties are actually meted out could either reinforce or erode such fear. **The committee recommends that future research examine how social stigma for acts of violence against women is generated and either sustained or eroded; such research would inform the development of more effective policies and programs.**

Formation of Perceptions of the Risk of Sanctions. There is a large body of research analyzing the links between perceptions of the risk of sanctions and behavior. However, very little is known about how such perceptions are formed. **The committee recommends that research be conducted on how perceptions of the risk of sanctions are generated and sustained over time for offenders who victimize women. Better studies are also needed of the effects of the crime rate on actual sanction levels and of how those effects in turn influence the formation of perceptions of the risk of punishment. Finally, it is important to explore Sherman's theory that initial deterrence (e.g., through arrest) can be made permanent by continually experimenting with novel police strategies, deployments, or enforcement priorities.**

How Responses to Crime Vary Across Time and Space. While some policies may be amenable to credible estimates of their average deterrent effects (e.g., the effects of arrest policies on intimate-partner violence), the capacity to translate those effects into predictions for specific places or populations is limited. **The committee urges research on the extent to which levels of violence against women respond to policy in specific cities or states rather than research on the average response across all cities and states.**

Links Between Intended and Actual Policy. Finally, the link between intended and actual policy has not been well explored. **The committee recommends that research examine how sanctions are generated and implemented so their effects on crime and on perceptions of the risk of sanctions can be better understood.**

1

Introduction

In January 2002, a committee of the National Research Council (NRC) convened a workshop to formulate a research agenda for addressing the continuing problem of violence against women. The findings and recommendations emerging from the workshop are presented in this report.

CONTEXT

Violence against women is a long-standing social problem in the United States and throughout the world. A recent survey on the prevalence and incidence of violence against women in the United States revealed that one in every six women has experienced an attempted or completed rape as a child and/or adult. Each year more than 300,000 women are forcibly raped, and more than 4 million suffer an aggravated or simple assault (Tjaden and Thoennes, 2000). The Bureau of Justice Statistics reports that between 1976 and 1999, murders of women accounted for 24 percent of total homicides in the United States. Approximately one-third of these victims were killed by a spouse, boyfriend, or other family member. Moreover, while homicides declined during the 1990s for both men and women, the decline in intimate-partner homicides was greater for male than for female victims (Fox and Zawitz, 2002).

The importance of the problem of violence against women was acknowledged by Congress with the passage of the Violence Against Women Act of 1994. The act included a mandate that the National Institute of Justice (NIJ) task the NRC with developing a research agenda to increase understanding and control of violence against women. In 1996, the NRC published the results of that study in *Understanding Violence Against Women*. The NRC report draws attention to the importance of building knowledge about violence against women and its prevention to support and inform national (and international) efforts to create a safer society for women and girls. It identifies a framework for conducting research in three areas: improving research methods, building knowledge about violence against women, and preventing violence against women. It also calls for developing a new federal infrastructure for conducting research on this important topic. In 1998, Congress provided new funds to NIJ for the implementation of some of these research recommendations. In addition to creating a program of studies under the NRC framework, NIJ, in partnership with the Office of Justice Programs' (OJP) Violence Against Women Office, initiated a significant program for evaluating criminal justice responses to violence against women. Box 1-1 summarizes activities and research conducted by OJP and NIJ under the Violence Against Women Act; Table 1-1, which appears at the end of the chapter,

---

BOX 1-1. Activities Under the Violence Against Women Act

In the first 5 years of implementation of the Violence Against Women Act, Congress appropriated about $1.6 billion for local initiatives and for process evaluations; in 1998, $5.5 million was earmarked for research. In October 2000, Congress authorized $3.3 billion over a 5-year period in the reauthorization of the act. The funds were to be used for the following major purposes:

- The continuation of S.T.O.P. Violence Against Women formula grants, including funding for state coalitions against sexual assault
- Rape prevention and education
- Fighting violence against women on college campuses
- Assistance for prosecutors to track down domestic abusers
- Expansion of shelters for battered women and their children

The reauthorization expanded the scope of the act on a few fronts, including education on violence against immigrant and disabled women and protections for such special populations. Funds also were set aside for such purposes as providing legal assistance for victims of sexual assault and domestic violence, and reviewing and expanding programs for sexual assault nurse examiners.

At the workshop, David Ford presented findings from his recent evaluation of the impact of the Violence Against Women Act. Ford and col-

presents NIJ-funded research projects in this area up to the end of 2000, organized under each of the major research recommendations of the NRC report (Note: the table does not include research funded by other government agencies in response to the recommendations in Understanding Violence Against Women).

One emphasis of the framework set forth in *Understanding Violence Against Women* is the need to improve research methods. The report calls for the use of clearly defined terms, particularly when delineating expected outcomes in evaluation studies, and for the development and validation of operational definitions and tools for measuring violence against women. NIJ has funded a handful of studies that evaluate measurement instruments (see Table 1-1), and also sponsored a workshop on measurement on November 20, 2000. To date, however, studies have not specifically addressed problems of definition as a main goal.

The report also recommends that national and community-level surveys include information on behavior, injuries, and other consequences of violence in measurements of the incidence and prevalence of violence

leagues (2002) found that the legislation has stimulated and supported both interventions to prevent violence against women and research to evaluate these interventions. NIJ has mounted a research program that follows both the mandates of the act and, to the extent possible, the recommendations of *Understanding Violence Against Women* (see Table 1-1). In general, the new federal funds available under the act have made violence against women a more productive and rewarding topic for many researchers.

However, funding for such research remains inadequate and thinly distributed. This is the case largely because of the high cost of both the rigorous methodologies, such as prospective (longitudinal) designs, necessary to understand the causes of violence against women and the experimental studies needed to identify the effects of various program efforts. In general, funds under the Violence Against Women Act have not been used to evaluate new policies or examine the underlying causes of violence against women.

Finally, we emphasize that research of the sort addressed in this report is not an abstract activity; it is directly related to and supportive of the responses of the criminal justice, health, and social service systems to violence against women. It is also informed by the scholarship that has come before it, much of which can be traced directly to the funding provided by Congress to NIJ. The outcomes of this research, in combination with assessments of the work in the field by the scholars who participated in the workshop, provided a critical backdrop to the recommendations offered in this report.

against women. It calls for more research on the social, cultural, and individual context and experience of violence in women's lives and on the results of this violence, including intergenerational consequences and costs to society. In addition, the report stresses the need for longitudinal studies tracing the developmental trajectory of violence against women and other violent behaviors.

In response to these recommendations, NIJ has funded many studies to examine the context of violence against women, particularly studies examining economic distress, race/ethnicity, and alcohol and drug abuse. No new longitudinal studies on this topic have been undertaken in the United States, however. The Dunedin Health and Development study (Moffitt et al., 2001) in New Zealand is an example of a population-based longitudinal study that has provided useful information about violence against women. Moreover, although support has been provided for selected studies on the consequences of violence against women, the need remains to measure the causes and consequences of violence against women in national and community surveys.

To build knowledge about preventing violence against women, the NRC report recommends that evaluation studies of prevention programs describe current services for victims and measure both short- and long-term effects of those services. It also recommends randomized, controlled outcome studies of legal and social service interventions with offenders, studies on the service-seeking behavior of victims, and studies on the use of discretion by officials in the criminal and civil justice systems. Although NIJ has funded many evaluation studies, evaluations of primary prevention programs—particularly educational programs—using experimental methods are still needed to measure long-term effects, as well as effects on the rate of new cases of violence against women. Similarly, few outcome studies of offender treatment use rigorous designs or measure long-term effects. There is also limited research on the effects of legal reforms on rates of reporting, arrests, and conviction, and little or no research on more recent legislative changes, such as sex offender notification laws, sexually violent predator laws, and laws criminalizing the use of "date rape drugs." NIJ has funded a few studies addressing service-seeking behavior, with a focus on minority women; police officer perceptions of domestic violence; and judicial and prosecutorial decisions regarding domestic and sexual violence cases (see Table 1-1).

WORKSHOP ON ISSUES IN RESEARCH ON VIOLENCE AGAINST WOMEN

Given the continuing nature of the problem of violence against women and the persisting gaps in research on the problem and its control,

Congress in 2000 asked the NRC to develop a detailed research agenda based on the recommendations of *Understanding Violence Against Women*. To address this new mandate, the NRC appointed a steering committee of four distinguished scholars and issued the following charge:

> A sub-committee of the Committee on Law and Justice will organize a workshop, bringing together researchers from various disciplines, including psychology, sociology, criminology, public health, statistics, epidemiology, and law, and policy officials from the Department of Justice and the Centers for Disease Control and Prevention. Among the social scientists will be those who have studied the victimization and perpetration of violence against women. This workshop will build upon the groundwork laid by the NRC Panel on Research on Violence Against Women, determining what progress has been made since the panel's report and what work still needs to be done, and recommending a new research agenda based on those determinations.
>
> The presentations and discussions at the workshop will focus on the following issues:
>
> - Trends and patterns of victimization
> - Violence across the life course
> - Spatial distributions of violence against women
> - Situational determinants of violence against women
> - Testing deterrence models
> - Assessment and development of primary prevention
> - Motivations of offenders, and implications for treatment
>
> Background papers will be commissioned and will be circulated before the workshop, where short presentations will lead to detailed discussions of the major areas to be explored. After the workshop, the subcommittee will meet to discuss the outcomes and reach consensus on recommendations. A summary of the meeting and the subcommittee's recommendations of steps to fill in research gaps will be prepared and submitted to the sponsor and other participants and interested parties.

In January 2002, with funds from NIJ, the steering committee, under the auspices of the NRC's Committee on Law and Justice, convened the Workshop on Issues in Research on Violence Against Women. The purpose of the workshop was to review the knowledge base that has emerged in this area since the publication of *Understanding Violence Against Women*—focusing particularly, but not exclusively, on studies completed between 1995 and 2000—and identify further research needs.

The steering committee commissioned eight papers by prominent researchers, identified scholars to serve as formal commentators, and invited a group of distinguished researchers and practitioners to participate in the 2-day workshop. The papers summarized important domains of research on violence against women, including prevalence and incidence, data sources, prevention and deterrence, and treatment for offenders (see Appendix C for a list of the commissioned papers). Following presentation of the papers, workshop participants discussed research gaps and suggested new efforts to meet research needs, especially to inform prevention strategies and assess intervention efforts. In general, this report is a synthesis of the presentations and the expertise of participants. The committee notes that a number of studies published between 1995 and 2000 were not covered by workshop papers or discussion. References for some of these studies are provided in an addendum to the reference list for the reader's information.

KEY THEMES

Before proceeding, we wish to emphasize an important theme that emerged from the committee's deliberations on the workshop papers and discussion. Because so little research on violence against women was conducted in the past, most such research has been conducted in isolation from the larger body of work on violence in general (including research such as that on violence by men, on violence by adolescents, and on criminal careers). This intellectual separation of research on violence against women also stems from the premise that distinctive features of the social and political context of such violence, particularly the context of intimate relationships, set it apart from other forms of violence. That is, women's greater exposure and vulnerability to attacks by intimates and greater probability of being injured in such attacks make violence against women distinctive. This distinction is an important one: female murder victims are eight times more likely to be killed by an intimate than are male murder victims, and women are the primary victims of stalking (Tjaden and Thoennes, 2000; Rennison, 2003).

The steering committee is nevertheless troubled by the almost total separation that has characterized this field. While there is dissimilarity in the contexts and outcomes of victimization for women and men, the committee questions whether behavioral patterns or causes of violent behavior are different enough to warrant this degree of separation. At this point in its development, a greater degree of integration of research on violence against and by women with the larger literature on crime and violence would enrich the former research intellectually and extend the lessons that can be learned about violence against women. Findings from research on violence against women could in turn be used to inform research on other types of violence. For example, in their analysis focusing on family homicide, Petrie and Garner (1990) identify characteristics that may help predict homicide and possibly other kinds of violence.

This conclusion is based on the observation that a substantial proportion of that violence occurs outside of intimate relationships. For example, the National Crime Victimization Survey found that approximately 38 percent of nonfatal violent crimes against women in 1994 were committed by a stranger (Craven, 1997). In 2000, the same survey again found that about one-third of all female victims of violent crime and one-third of rape and sexual assault victims described the offender as a stranger (Rennison, 2001).

At this point, we have no evidence that a separate theory is needed to explain violence by intimates and no reason to expect that the closeness (or distance) of the relationship between victim and offender sets the conditions for theoretical predictions of violent offending. For example, Holtzworth-Munroe and Meehan (2002) describe a batterer typology (see Chapter 5) that uses the broader literature on delinquency and violent behavior to show that batterers can be classified according to generality of violence (i.e., marital only or extrafamilial). This typology includes a subtype of generally violent/antisocial batterers whose marital violence is conceptualized as part of their general use of aggression and engagement in antisocial behavior.[1] Moreover, a growing body of empirical evidence demonstrates that perpetrators of violence against women commonly have histories of violence and conduct problems outside of intimate relationships (Giordano et al., 1999; Capaldi and Clark, 1998; Farrington, 1994). On the basis of this evidence, Moffitt et al. (2001:175) conclude:

> . . . childhood conduct problems, even when measured in the first decade of life, foretell relationship violence equally well in the adult lives of both males and females.
>
> The finding that young people who have a history of antisocial conduct problems are likely to employ similar aggressive tactics later in their primary adult relationships suggests the hypothesis that the causes of conduct disorder may also be at the root causes of partner violence. Interventions conceptualized as treatments for conduct problems gain even more urgency if they are re-conceptualized as primary prevention for future domestic violence.

It is noteworthy that this conclusion is not limited to male perpetrators. Moffitt et al. (2001) argue convincingly that women perpetrate much violence in the context of intimate relationships that is not purely defensive, though at much lower rates of frequency and severity than men. Thus, it is important to expand both theoretical and empirical models to

---

[1]Felson (2002) also suggests studying motives for violence against women within a framework of motivations for violence in general.

better understand female-perpetrated violence, the contexts in which it occurs, and its consequences for both victims and offenders.

Discussion in the remaining chapters of this report, then, reflects the committee's view that, to a somewhat greater extent than is currently the case, studies of violence against women should draw upon the larger literature. The theoretical and longitudinal literatures on violent crime and aggression generally are especially pertinent in this regard for determining whether new longitudinal studies focused on women's violent victimization are needed.

Finally, because the majority of extant research on violence against women addresses intimate-partner violence, much of this report has a similar focus. The committee notes, however, that over two-thirds of homicides against women take place outside of this context, and that violence against women is perpetrated by strangers and acquaintances. Therefore, the committee believes the research agenda of the federal government on violence against women should be expanded to include these other cases. Further, the exploration of women's violent victimization during the workshop included their own violent acts. As with violent victimization of women, violence by women may differ from that by men in important ways, specifically with regard to its context and correlates. As more than one participant made clear at the workshop, in many cases violence *by* women can be understood only in the context of violence committed *against* women. It may be useful to consider a framework whereby these different types of violence in which women play roles, as either offenders or victims, are connected.

REPORT ORGANIZATION

The remainder of this report is divided into six chapters. Chapter 2 reviews the means researchers have available for measuring violence against women and the knowledge thus obtained. Chapter 3 addresses the social and geographic factors that determine the social ecological risks of violence against women. Chapter 4 presents what is known about prevention and deterrence. Chapter 5 examines means for identifying and treating offenders. Finally, Chapter 6 prioritizes the key points and recommendations made throughout the report.

TABLE 1-1 NIJ-Funded Research on Violence Against Women, by
Recommendations of NRC Report, 1995–2000

Principal Investigator, Project Title	Method	Level	Project Goal
Recommendation 1: Researchers and practitioners should more clearly define the terms used in their work.			
Recommendation 2: Research funds should be made available for the development and validation of scales and other tools for the measurement of violence against women to make operational key and most used definitions. The development process should include input from subpopulations with whom the instrument will be used, for example, people of color or specific ethnic groups.			
Campbell, J. C., Risk Factors for Homicide in Violent Intimate Relationships	Analysis of official records	Multicity	Evaluate the Danger Assessment Instrument; identify risk factors preceding intimate-partner homicide.
O'Sullivan, C., Field Testing Domestic Violence Risk Assessment Instruments: A Planning Study for an Experimental Evaluation	Evaluation		Evaluate the validity and reliability of instruments being used to assess a domestic abuse victim's level of risk, with a focus on the Mosaic-20.
Campbell, J. C., Intimate Risk Violence Assessment Instruments: A Prospective Validation Field Experiment	Evaluation: interviews, analysis of criminal records	Multicity	Evaluate the effectiveness of four extant risk assessment instruments: Mosaic-20, Danger Assessment, Domestic Violence Screening Instrument, and Kingston-Screening Instrument for Domestic Violence.
Cook, S., Investigating the Roles of Context, Meaning, and Method in the Measurement of Central Violence Against Women Constructs	Survey, interview		Review measurement instruments and research practices in research on violence against women; determine the prevalence of violence-against-women constructs, and develop a new model; explore use of computer-based data collection for research on violence against women in correctional and health care settings.

Continued

TABLE 1-1 Continued

Principal Investigator, Project Title	Method	Level	Project Goal

Recommendation 3: National and community-level representative sample survey studies using the most valid instrumentation and questioning techniques available to measure incidence and prevalence of violence against women are needed. These studies should collect data not only on behavior, but also on injuries and other consequences of violence. Studies of incidence and prevalence of perpetration of violence against women are also needed. National and community surveys of other topics, such as women's mental or physical health or social or economic well-being, should be encouraged to include questions pertaining to violence against women. Furthermore, identification and secondary analysis of existing datasets with respect to violence against women should be funded.

Principal Investigator, Project Title	Method	Level	Project Goal
Fisher, B., Extent and Nature of Sexual Victimization of College Women	Survey	National	Measure the prevalence of sexual victimization.
Tjaden, P., Violence and Threats of Violence Against Women in America	Survey	National	Measure the prevalence and incidence of rape, physical assault, and stalking.
Weiss, H., A Population-Based Comparison of Assaultive Injury Patterns Among Hospitalized Pregnant Women Compared to Women of Reproductive Age	Analysis of existing dataset	Multistate	Measure the incidence of assault among hospitalized pregnant women; develop a mechanism to measure the burden and trends of serious violence against pregnant women.
Fagan, J., and Wilt, S., Social and Neighborhood Risks of Violence Towards Women: Implications for Prevention	Analysis of existing dataset	Community	Examine the spatial distribution of violence against women in New York City; estimate risk factors.
Wells, W., An Analysis of Unexamined Issues in the Intimate-Partner Homicide Decline: Race, Quality of Victim Services, Offender Accountability, and System Accountability	Analysis of existing dataset	State	Analyze rates of intimate-partner homicide by race and gender of victims and offenders; test how support services, offender accountability, and system accountability affect victim safety.

TABLE 1-1 Continued

Principal Investigator, Project Title	Method	Level	Project Goal
Salomon, A., Secondary Data Analysis on the Etiology, Course, and Consequences of Intimate-Partner Violence Against Extremely Poor Women	Analysis of existing longitudinal dataset	Community	Measure rates of lifetime adult-partner violence and childhood abuse.

Recommendation 4: All research on violence against women should take into account the context within which women live their lives and in which the violence occurs. This context should include the broad social and cultural context, as well as individual factors. Work should include more qualitative research, such as ethnographic research, as well as quantitative research, designed to uncover the confluence of factors such as race, socioeconomic status, age, and sexual orientation in shaping the context and experience of violence in women's lives.

Benson, M., Economic Distress, Community Context and Intimate Violence	Analysis of existing dataset	National	Examine the effect of economic distress on violence against women.
Jasinski, J. L., Violence Against Women: An Examination of Developmental Antecedents Among Black, Caucasian, and Hispanic Women	Analysis of existing dataset	National	Examine the developmental antecedents of violence against women by race/ethnicity.
Malcoe, L. H., Understanding Partner Violence in Native American Women	Interview, survey	Community	Measure the prevalence of intimate-partner violence among Native American women in Plains tribes; examine risk and protective factors.
Perilla, J., Domestic Abuse Among Latinos: Description and Intervention		Community	Explore patterns of abuse within the context of Latino cultural values.
Pennell, S., Examining the Nature and Correlates of Domestic Violence Among Female Arrestees in San Diego	Interview	Community	Examine the incidence and prevalence of domestic violence among female arrestees and the relationship among alcohol and drugs, violent victimization, and service and treatment needs of female offenders.

Continued

TABLE 1-1 Continued

Principal Investigator, Project Title	Method	Level	Project Goal
Downs, W., Alcohol Problems and Violence Against Women	Interview	Multisite	Describe the association between alcohol abuse and domestic violence among women in alcohol treatment programs and women receiving services for domestic violence victimization.
Richie, B., Understanding the Link Between Violence Against Women and Women's Participation in Crime	Survey, life history interviews	State	Examine experiences with violence against women among incarcerated women.
LeRoy, B. W., A Michigan Study on Women with Physical Disabilities	Survey	State	Determine the extent of and risk factors for domestic violence among women with disabilities.
Brush, L., Qualitative Research on Battering, Work and Welfare	Interview, participant observation	Community	Examine the timing of battering as women transition from welfare to work, and the effect of battering on women's work, relationships, and welfare recipiency.
Block, C. R., Risk of Serious Injury or Death in Intimate Violence	Interview	Community	Identify risk factors of battered women for serious injury or death.
Jumper Thurman, P., Research on Violence Against Indian Women: Community Readiness and Intervention	Phone interviews, focus groups	Community	Compare prevention resources, cultural norms, and community climate regarding violence against women among Native American communities.
Peacock, T., Community-Based Institutional Assessment to Reduce Risk of Continued Abuse to Native American Women	Evaluation (audit)	Community	Examine how safety needs of Native American women are or are not addressed by the criminal justice system.

TABLE 1-1 Continued

Principal Investigator, Project Title	Method	Level	Project Goal
Senturia, K., Cultural Issues Affecting Domestic Violence Services in Ethnic and Hard-to-Reach Populations	Qualitative	Community	Examine satisfaction with domestic violence services and the cultural experience of domestic violence among women from eight ethnic groups and the lesbian/ bisexual/transsexual community.
Krishnan, S., Understanding Domestic Violence in Multi-Ethnic Rural Communities: A Focus on Collaboration Among the Courts, Law Enforcement Agencies, and the Shelters	Survey, interview, life histories	Community	Examine service-seeking and services offered for the shelter, law enforcement, and court systems, with a focus on minority women and those in rural or underserved communities.
Erez, E., Violence Against Immigrant Women and Systematic Responses: An Exploratory Study	Interview, survey	Multistate	Examine the experience of violence among immigrant women and systematic responses to immigrant battered women.
Soriano, F., A Comparison of Partner Violence in Latino Communities: Migrant Workers, Immigrants, Non-immigrants	Survey	Community	Measure the prevalence of intimate-partner violence among nonmigrant or seasonal worker U.S.-born Latinas, nonmigrant or seasonal worker immigrant Latinas, and migrant or seasonal worker Latinas; examine cultural and other factors.
Magen, R., Violence Against Athabascan Native Women in the Copper River Basin	Survey, interview	Community	Examine the cultural context and the nature and extent of violence against women among Athabascan Native Alaskans.
Rodriguez, R., Community Partnership Models Addressing Violence Against Migrant and Seasonal Farmworker Women	Survey, interview, focus groups	Multisite	Compare grassroots and agency-based models of domestic violence outreach/ education, and use of the criminal justice system for migrant and seasonal farmworker women.

Continued

TABLE 1-1 Continued

Principal Investigator, Project Title	Method	Level	Project Goal
Worden, A., Beliefs and Perceptions About Domestic Violence: Effects on Individual, Contextual, and Community Factors	Telephone interviews	State	Measure attitudes, values, and perceptions regarding domestic violence, and their relationship with perceptions about interventions and sanctions.
Raymond, J., Sex Trafficking of Women in Five Regional Cities	Interview	Multicity	Examine the circumstances of immigrant and U.S. women in the sex industry, including experiences with emotional and physical abuse.
Malcoe, L. H., Partner Drug and Alcohol Use, Mediating Factors, and Violence Against Women	Survey	Community	Examine the effects of women's and men's drug and alcohol abuse on intimate-partner violence among arrestees for drug offenses.
Dutton, M., Ecological Model of Battered Women's Experience over Time	Interview, longitudinal	Multisite	Describe patterns of battered women's experience over time; test a prediction model of change in abuse; examine risk reduction strategies of battered women.
Myers, S., The Effects of Welfare Recipiency on Domestic Violence	Analysis of existing dataset	National	Examine the effects of welfare recipiency on domestic violence.
Block, C. R., Does Community Crime Prevention Make a Difference Behind Closed Doors?	Analysis of existing dataset	Community	Examine the effect of community norms on violence against women

Recommendation 5: Longitudinal research, with particular attention to developmental and life-span perspectives, should be undertaken to study the developmental trajectory of violence against women and whether and how it differs from the development of other violent behaviors. Particular attention should be paid to factors associated with the initial development of violent behavior, its maintenance, escalation, or dimunition over time, and the influence of socioeconomic, cultural, and ethnic factors. Funding is encouraged for identification and analysis of existing datasets that include relevant information. In addition, research on the causes and consequences of violent behavior should include questions about violence against women.

TABLE 1-1 Continued

Principal Investigator, Project Title	Method	Level	Project Goal
King, L., and King, D., Male-Perpetrated Domestic Violence: Testing a Series of Multifactorial Family Models	Analysis of existing dataset	National	Examine factors contributing to male-perpetrated domestic violence and effects on partners' mental health and the behavior of offspring.
Loftin, C., Investigating Intimate-Partner Violence Using NIBRS Data	Analysis of existing dataset	National	Examine correlates and causes of intimate-partner homicide; compare patterns across communities.
Moffitt, T., Developmental Antecedents of Partner Violence	Analysis of longitudinal database	New Zealand	Examine the prevalence of physical abuse and risk factors for perpetrators and victims.
Jouriles, E. N., Development of Violence Against Women	Analysis of existing dataset	National	Examine developmental antecendents of violence against women.
Mazerolle, P., Developmental Theory and Battering Incidents: Examining the Relationship Between Discrete Offender Groups and Intimate-Partner Violence	Interview, analysis of official records	Community	Examine relationships between offender groups and intimate-partner violence, using developmental and life-span perspectives.
White, J., Developmental Antecedents of Violence Against Women: A Longitudinal Approach	Analysis of existing longitudinal dataset	National	Examine the developmental antecedents of violence against young women among a college student population, examining perpetration and victimization.
McDonald, R., Domestic Violence and Child Aggression			Examine the relationship between exposure of children to domestic violence and children's aggressive behavior.

Recommendation 6: Research is needed on the consequences of violence against women that includes intergenerational consequences and costs to society, including lost productivity and the use of the criminal justice, medical, and social service systems. Such research should address the effects of race and socioeconomic status on consequences of violence.

Continued

TABLE 1-1 Continued

Principal Investigator, Project Title	Method	Level	Project Goal
Coulter, M., The Relationship Between Welfare, Domestic Violence and Employment	Survey, interview, analysis of administrative data	State	Examine the impact of violence against women on the economic self-sufficiency of women welfare recipients.
Naylor Goodwin, S., Violence Against Women: The Role of Welfare Reform	Longitudinal cohort interview	County	Determine the impacts of domestic violence on employment, the impacts of welfare reform on women's experiences of domestic violence, and the effect of specific services on those impacts.
Bogat, G. A., Understanding the Intergenerational Transmission of Violence Against Women from Pregnancy Through the First Year of Life	Interview, longitudinal	Multisite	Examine the effect of battering of mothers on their infants during pregnancy and the first year of life.

Recommendation 7: Evaluations of preventive and treatment intervention efforts must clearly define the outcomes expected from the intervention. These outcome measures should derive from an explicit theory underlying each intervention. Defining outcomes requires close collaboration between researchers and service providers.

Recommendation 8: Programs designed to prevent sexual and intimate-partner violence should be subject to rigorous evaluation of both short- and long-term effects. Programs designed to prevent delinquency, substance abuse, teenage pregnancy, gang involvement, or general violence (including conflict mediation programs) should include evaluation of risk factors for and prevention of intimate and sexual violence. In addition, studies of at-risk children and adolescents should include an examination of the relationship of risk factors, such as poverty, childhood victimization, and brain injury, to outcomes of sexual and intimate-partner violence.

Heckert, A., Predicting Levels of Abuse and Reassault Among Batterer Program Participants	Analysis of existing longitudinal dataset	Multisite	Build a prediction model to identify risk factors and outcomes of arrested batterers.
Jouriles, E., Children of Battered Women: Reducing Risk for Abuse	Evaluation	Community	Examine intervention outcomes for mothers and children in reducing risk for child maltreatment.

TABLE 1-1 Continued

Principal Investigator, Project Title	Method	Level	Project Goal
Linares, L., The Effects of Community Violence on Women and Children	Dyad interviews, observation	Community	Examine the effect of community on family aggression related to maternal practices in high-crime neighborhoods.
Siegel, J. A., Risk Factors for Violent Victimization of Women: A Prospective Study	Analysis of existing dataset	Community	Examine child abuse as a risk factor for adult victimization.
Betts, P., Women's Experience with Violence: A Collaborative Research Initiative for the Center for Research on Women and the Memphis Sexual Assault Resource Center	Analysis of program and official records, interview	Community	Examine risk factors for sexual violence against women; evaluate a local sexual violence resource center.

Recommendation 9: Studies that describe current services for victims of violence and evaluate their effectiveness are needed. Studies to investigate the factors associated with victims' service-seeking behavior, including delaying seeking of services or not seeking services at all, are also needed. These studies should describe and evaluate innovative or alternative approaches or settings for identifying and providing services to victims of violence against women.

Resnick, H., Prevention of Post-Rape Psychopathology in Women	Evaluation	Community	Evaluate video-based preventive intervention.
Enos, V., An Intervention to Improve Documentation of Domestic Violence in Medical Records	Literature review, interview, focus groups, evaluation	City	Develop, implement, and evaluate a training intervention to improve documentation of abuse in health care settings.
Sullivan, C., Using a Longitudinal Dataset to Further Our Understanding of the Trajectory of Intimate Violence over Time	Evaluation, longitudinal	Community	Evaluate strengths-based intervention for victims of violence against women.
Weisz, A., An Evaluation of Family Advocacy with a Team Approach	Evaluation	Community	Evaluate victim advocate services.

Continued

TABLE 1-1 Continued

Principal Investigator, Project Title	Method	Level	Project Goal
Nagin, D., Dugan, L., and Rosenfeld, R., The Impact of Legal Advocacy on Intimate-Partner Homicide	Analysis of existing dataset	Multisite (48 cities)	Evaluate the impact of legal advocacy efforts on rates of intimate-partner homicide in terms of exposure-reducing potential.
Chaiken, M., Impact of VAWA: What Counts?	Case studies	Multisite	Assess the impact of funds provided under the Violence Against Women Act in addressing domestic violence (victim safety, offender accountability).
Isaac, N., Corporate Sector Response to Domestic Violence	Survey, interview, case study	National	Explore the responsiveness of the corporate sector to employees' experiences of domestic violence.
Bronson, D., Ramos, D., and Bohmer, C., An Evaluation of Victim Advocacy in Ohio	Evaluation	State	Describe and evaluate victim advocacy services in terms of personal functioning and pursuit of adjudication.
Ruch, L. O., Reporting Sexual Assault to the Police in Hawaii	Interview	State	Examine variables influencing the reporting of sexual violence to police.
Dutton, M., National Evaluation of the Rural Domestic and Child Victimization Enforcement Grant Program—Phase I and II	Evaluation	National	Evaluate this program designed to learn about domestic violence in rural families and increase the safety of rural abused women and children.
Alpert, G. P., The Lexington County Court: A Partnership and Evaluation	Evaluation	Community	Assess the impact of domestic violence court on victim safety, and the accountability of offenders and the court system.
Uekert, B., and Dupree, C., National Evaluation of Grants to Combat Violent Crimes Against Women on Campus	Evaluation	National	Document the impact of Violence Against Women Office (VAWO)–funded college campus programs on violence against women.

TABLE 1-1 Continued

Principal Investigator, Project Title	Method	Level	Project Goal
Ames, L., Evaluating Domestic Violence Programs in Clinton County	Evaluation	Community	Evaluate VAWO-funded programs to encourage arrest policies for domestic violence.
McDermott, M. J., Responding to Domestic Violence in Southern Illinois: An Evaluation Partnership	Evaluation	Community	Evaluate outcomes of a VAWO-funded pro-arrest project.
Ryan, R., Evaluation of Protective Order Enforcement Team (POET)	Evaluation–comparative analysis	State	Assess and compare the effectiveness of POET and Domestic Assault Response Team.
McFarlane, J., Increasing Victim Safety and System Accountability with Protection Orders: Evaluating a Collaborative Intervention Between Health Care and Criminal Justice	Evaluation	County	Implement and test an advocacy case management intervention in the specialized district attorney's office that aims to inform victims about how they can obtain protection orders and to offer advice and support regarding safety, emotional well-being, and work productivity.
Whitcomb, D., and Fisher, B., Research on Procedures of Institutions of Higher Education to Report Sexual Assaults	Survey, content analysis of official documents	National	Describe policies and procedures of institutions of higher education for responding to reports of sexual assaults.
Burt, M., National Impact Evaluation of Victim Services Programs Funded Through the S.T.O.P. Violence Against Women Formula Program	Evaluation	National	Describe the variety of S.T.O.P.-funded victim service programs, the community and state contexts in which they operate, and their effect on victim outcomes; assess the degree to which S.T.O.P. funding for victim service programs has affected program services, community context, and victim outcomes.

Continued

TABLE 1-1 Continued

Principal Investigator, Project Title	Method	Level	Project Goal
Uekert, B., and McEwen, T., National Evaluation of the Arrest Policies Program Under the Violence Against Women Act	Evaluation	National	Explore local implementations of model programs; study interactions among officials to develop a model of collaboration for a systematic approach to domestic violence; assess program effectiveness; and identify innovative, unique, and promising projects.
Luna, E., Impact Evaluation of the S.T.O.P. Grant Programs for Reducing Violence Against Women	Impact evaluation, case study	National	Evaluate programs funded under the S.T.O.P. Violence Against Indian Women grants to understand the cultural and legal context of reducing violence against women among Indian tribes; evaluate the impact of tribal programs to reduce violence against women; and make recommendations for improving existing programs and developing new programs for tribes to reduce violence against women.
Pennell, S., The Nature and Scope of Violence Against Women in San Diego	Review of records	Community	Describe characteristics of victims, batterers, and domestic violence incidents using data from emergency shelters and police records.
Uchida, C., Evaluating the DVERT program in Colorado Springs	Process evaluation	Community	Examine the intervention process of the Colorado Springs Domestic Violence Enhanced Response Team (DVERT).
Connors, E., National Evaluation of the Domestic Violence Victims' Civil Legal Assistance (CLA) Program	Evaluation	National	Describe types of problems being addressed and projects being supported; examine how CLA programs assess need and conduct outreach to clients; and examine immediate and long-term impacts on clients.

TABLE 1-1 Continued

Principal Investigator, Project Title	Method	Level	Project Goal
Recommendation 10: Randomized, controlled outcome studies are needed to identify the program and community features that account for the effectiveness of legal or social service interventions with various groups of offenders.			
Havens, C., Evaluation of Special Session Domestic Violence: Enhanced Advocacy and Interventions	Evaluation		Evaluate the effectiveness of specialized domestic violence court sessions in terms of victim safety and offender recidivism.
Eckhardt, C., Stages and Processes of Change and Associated Treatment Outcomes in Partner Assaultive Men	Evaluation	Community	Examine the effects of court-referred batterer intervention programs on subsequent attrition and recidivism.
Lyon, E., Impact Evaluation of a Special Session Domestic Violence: Enhanced Advocacy and Interventions	Evaluation	Community	Evaluate outcomes of a program for male domestic violence offenders.
Hartley, C., The Cook County Court Target Abuser Call (TAC): An Evaluation of a Specialized Domestic Violence Court	Evaluation	Community	Examine the effect of a specialized domestic violence court on conviction rates, victim appearance rates, etc.
Davis, R., The Brooklyn Domestic Violence Experiment	Experimental design	Community	Determine the effect of court-mandated batterer treatment in Brooklyn in terms of reoffending and attitude change.
Feder, L., A Test of the Efficacy of Court-Mandated Counseling for Domestic Violence Offenders	Experimental design	County	Test the effectiveness of court-mandated counseling in reducing repeat violence.
Greenspan, R., and Weisburd, D., The Richmond/Police Foundation Domestic Violence Partnership	Experimental design	Community	Test the effects of social workers who provide crisis intervention on the scene of domestic violence incidents, as well as follow-up services.

Continued

TABLE 1-1 Continued

Principal Investigator, Project Title	Method	Level	Project Goal

Recommendation 11: Studies are needed that examine discretionary processes in the criminal and civil justice systems, including implementation of new laws and reforms, charging and prosecutorial decision making, jury decision making, and judicial decision making. Legal research, which supplies the theoretical basis behind legal interpretations and reforms, is also needed.

Principal Investigator, Project Title	Method	Level	Project Goal
Hotaling, G., and Buzawa, E., Criminal Justice Intervention in Domestic Violence: Victim Preferences, Victim Satisfaction and Factors Impacting on Revictimization	Analysis of existing dataset	Community	Examine risk factors for victims and perpetrators, and preferences and dissatisfaction of victims with regard to the criminal justice system.
Belknap, J., A Longitudinal Study of Battered Women in the System: The Victims' and Decision Makers' Perceptions	Interviews, longitudinal	Multisite	Examine victim and prosecutor perceptions of the problem, and influences on decisions of battered women who have gone through the court system.
Rivara, F., Protection of Women: Health and Justice Outcomes	Follow-up evaluation	Community	Examine the effects of protection orders.
Smith, B., An Evaluation of Efforts to Implement No-Drop Policies: Two Central Values in Conflict	Evaluation	Multisite	Evaluate the effects of no-drop policies.
Finn, M., Evaluation of Policies, Procedures, and Programs Addressing Violence Against Women	Evaluation	Multisite	Evaluate the effects of no-drop policies.
Burt, M., and Harrell, A., National Evaluation of the VAWA Grants	Evaluation	National	Document grant activities and programs under the Violence Against Women Act; assess outcomes and accomplishments of grantees.
Wolf, M. E., Protection of Women: Health and Justice Outcomes	Evaluation, cohort study	Community	Evaluate the effectiveness of protection orders.

TABLE 1-1 Continued

Principal Investigator, Project Title	Method	Level	Project Goal
Keilitz, S., Domestic Violence Courts: Jurisdiction, Organization, Performance Goals and Measures	Survey, interview	National	Provide a comprehensive list of domestic violence courts; develop performance goals.
Sviridoff, M., King's County Felony Domestic Court Research Partnership: Exploring Implementation and Early Impacts	Evaluation	County	Evaluate a county domestic violence court.
Giacomazzi, A., and Smithey, M., Violence Against Women in the City of El Paso, Texas: Developing Research–Practitioner Partnerships	Evaluation	Community	Evaluate the effect of domestic violence training on police officer perceptions of domestic violence, the amount of time police officers spend on the scene with victims of domestic violence, and the number of cases accepted for prosecution and resulting in conviction.
McEwen, T., and Miller, N., Study of the Effectiveness of State Anti-Stalking Efforts and Legislation	Survey	National	Assess the status and effect of state antistalking efforts and laws.
McEwen, T., Impact Evaluation of S.T.O.P. Grants: Law Enforcement and Prosecution	Evaluation	Multisite	Evaluate the impact of a cross section of activities supported under the Law Enforcement and Prosecution purpose area of the S.T.O.P. formula grants.
Buzawa, E., Understanding, Preventing, and Controlling Domestic Violence Incidents	Interview	Community	Examine characteristics of domestic violence offenses, offenders, and victims in a proactive court setting.
Spohn, C., Prosecutors' Charging Decisions in Sexual Assault Cases	Analysis of official records	Multicity	Examine the effect of victim, suspect, and case characteristics on prosecutors' charging decisions.

Continued

TABLE 1-1 Continued

Principal Investigator, Project Title	Method	Level	Project Goal
Caliber Associates, Educational Development Center, National Center for State Courts, Evaluation of a Multi-Site Demonstration of Collaborations to Address Domestic Violence and Child Maltreatment	Evaluation	Multisite	Measure the extent to which collaboration of sites under the Green Book demonstration project resulted in system change and improvements in safety, repeat abuse, and batterer accountability.
Harrell, A., and Newmark, L., Evaluation of a Multi-Site Demonstration for Enhanced Judicial Oversight of Domestic Violence Cases	Evaluation	Multisite	Evaluate enhanced judicial oversight to determine the effect of victim services and strong judicial oversight of and graduated sanctions for domestic violence offenders on recidivism, defendant and system accountability, and victim safety.
Belknap, J., Factors Related to Domestic Violence Court Dispositions in Large Urban Areas	Interview, survey, analysis of official records	Community	Examine factors that influence judicial and prosecutorial decision making in domestic violence cases, and factors that influence victim/witness reluctance in bringing batterers to successful adjudication.
Worden, A., Models of Community Coordination in Response to Partner Violence	Survey, interview, observation, focus groups	State	Develop a typology of community coordination models, and assess their components and impact on victims' safety, perceptions of system effectiveness, revictimization, and satisfaction with responses.
Morrill, A. C., Child Custody and Visitation When the Father Batters the Mother	Evaluation	Multisite	Assess the impact of Model Code provisions regarding child custody and visitation and judicial knowledge of domestic violence issues.

TABLE 1-1 Continued

Principal Investigator, Project Title	Method	Level	Project Goal
Saccuzzo, D., Mandatory Custody Mediation Resulting in Formal Recommendations: A Window on Process and Outcome for Violent Families	Content analysis	Community	Compare child adjustment factors in violent and nonviolent families to determine whether group differences are reflected in custody and visitation plans; study custody decisions resulting from mandatory custody mediation; and evaluate custody decisions in terms of safety.
Isaac, N., Medical Records as Legal Evidence in Domestic Violence Cases	Review of medical records	Community	Describe, from a legal perspective, the documentation of domestic violence in abused women's medical charts.
Holt, V. L., History of Intimate-Partner Violence and the Determination of Custody and Visitation Among Couples Petitioning for Dissolution of Marriage	Analysis of police and court data	County	Examine the relationship between a history of intimate-partner violence and determination of child custody and visitation agreements among couples who filed for divorce.
Crandall, C., Impact Evaluation of a SANE [Sexual Assault Nurse Examiners] Unit in Albuquerque, New Mexico	Impact evaluation (quasi-experimental)	Community	Measure the impact of programs in law enforcement, prosecution, and health care services.
Ford, D., and Bachman, R., A Synthesis of the Research and Evaluation from the VAWA	Literature review	National	Review the state of knowledge on the impacts of justice components of the Violence Against Women Act to describe how the act has helped advance knowledge about effective controls.

Recommendation 12: The panel recommends that government agencies develop a coordinated strategy to strengthen the creation of a research base that is focused on prevention of violence against women and interventions for offenders and victims.

Continued

TABLE 1-1 Continued

Principal Investigator, Project Title	Method	Level	Project Goal

Recommendation 13: The panel recommends that a minimum of three to four research centers be established within academic or other appropriate settings to support the development of studies and training programs focused on violence against women, to provide mechanisms for collaboration between researchers and practitioners and technical assistance for integrating research into service provision.

Principal Investigator, Project Title	Method	Level	Project Goal
Worden, A., Research on Violence Against Women: Synthesis for Practitioners	Literature review	National	Synthesize research on violence against women to guide practitioners.

2

Nature and Scope of
Violence Against Women

As discussed in Chapter 1, the 1996 NRC report *Understanding Violence Against Women* outlines a series of methodological problems that have impeded the development of knowledge in this area. In the years since that report was produced, some of these problems have been addressed (e.g., the inclusion of questions about violence against women in surveys pertaining to other types of high-risk or violent behavior), yet others remain. This chapter focuses on the need for a coordinated and integrated research strategy that can build stronger scientific databases to enhance our understanding of violence against women.

Much of what is known about the violent victimization of women has been derived from methodologically disparate survey data. Certainly, survey research has been instrumental in setting some parameters for the scope of two types of violence—intimate-partner violence and sexual assault. Data on these problems indicate that the risk of such victimization varies substantially across racial and ethnic groups (Dugan and Apel, 2002; Rennison and Welchans, 2000; Tjaden and Thoennes, 1998). Nevertheless, survey research has been less successful in providing reliable estimates of the prevalence and incidence of intimate-partner violence and sexual assault, about the context of these violent events, about the developmental patterns of such violence over time, and about the ways in which women's victimization experiences may be linked to women's offending behaviors (Campbell et al., 2002a; Richie, 1996). To advance a more systematic approach to the study of violence against women, this chapter considers in turn the strengths and weaknesses of the major national datasets that provide information on violence against women; other datasets that were not designed to examine violent victimization, but have included relevant questions pertaining to the violent victimization of women; information provided by current datasets about the extent and nature of violence against women; and methodological issues that have precluded linking extant datasets, improving measurement, and enhancing ongoing survey research.

MAJOR DATASETS

A wide array of datasets provides information on violence against adult and/or adolescent females, although this is not always the primary focus of the various data collection efforts. Many of these datasets include information from national samples of women or large groups of U.S. women that are representative of a particular population. Each has both strengths and limitations. The most serious limitations of existing datasets are as follows: (1) most were designed for primary purposes other than collecting information on violence against women; (2) most are not continuous and so cannot show changes over time; and (3) although many collect data on similar issues (e.g., prevalence), definitions of violence against women, as well as data collection instruments, vary, making it difficult to compare results. These and other shortcomings, especially nonresponse and false-response errors, need to be addressed in future research. At a 1998 conference on research on violence against women, sponsored by the Centers for Disease Control and Prevention (CDC) and the National Institute of Justice (NIJ), a matrix of datasets that include some information on violence against women was created with an eye to determining how to link information from disparate surveys, an issue discussed further below. The committee has expanded this matrix somewhat and included it here as Table 2-1. In a paper commissioned for the workshop, Campbell et al. (2002a) describe the following major datasets on which most researchers in the field currently rely:

The National Crime Victimization Survey (NCVS), sponsored by the Bureau of Justice Statistics (BJS), is the second-largest ongoing government-run U.S. survey (Bachman, 2000). It is the most extensive victimization data source, documenting characteristics of victims and nonvictims aged 12 and older living within sampled housing units. In addition to detailed information on each household and the interviewed individual within that household, the survey documents respondents' recent experiences as crime victims, including details of each event and its consequences. From 1972 to the present, data collection, using a rotating panel design in selected housing units, has been conducted seven times during each 3-year period.[1] In 2000, the response rate was 93.0 percent of eligible households and 89.3 percent of eligible individuals (Rennison, 2002). This survey is one of only a handful of continuous datasets that collects information on violence against women. Each year, BJS uses the data to publish reports on current crime distributions and to document patterns and consequences for several types of victims (Bureau of Justice Statistics, 2000).

NCVS data do permit an examination of whether and how violent victimization differs for women and men, but they have several limitations. While the redesign effort in 1992 led to improved estimates of domestic and sexual violence (see Bachman and Taylor, 1994, for a thorough description of the redesign effort and its improvements), analysis of long-term trends has been curtailed because the content of assault and sexual assault items was changed. In addition, no information is collected on victimization history and the communities and cultures within which the violence occurs, although NCVS data with census-tract codes attached are available to researchers with permission from the U.S. Census Bureau. Data pertaining to the immediate context of violent events (e.g., urban setting, home ownership, public housing) are also limited.

The National Surveys of Family Violence (NSFV) encompassed two cross-sectional surveys conducted by the University of New Hampshire under the auspices of the Family Violence Research Program, sponsored by the National Institute of Mental Health (Gelles and Straus, 1988; Straus et al., 1988): the first was conducted in 1975 and relied on in-person home interviews; the second was conducted in 1985 and relied on random-digital-dial telephone interviews. Each was designed to provide a comprehensive examination of violence in the family, including spouse abuse, child abuse (including physical punishment as a form of discipline), sibling-to-sibling abuse, and parent abuse (victimization of a parent or parents by the child/children of the family). The surveys were intended to provide data on the prevalence of these various types of family violence and to identify the risk (and protective) factors involved.

Family violence was operationalized with the Conflict Tactics Scales (CTS) (Straus, 1979). These scales are based on self-reports of 18 behaviors (grouped into three subscales consisting of rational, verbal, and violent acts) that may have occurred within the context of a disagreement. Over the course of the two surveys, the CTS were modified to include an additional series of questions regarding whether an act of violence produced an injury that required medical attention (Gelles, 1987).

These surveys represented the first nationwide examination of vio-

---

[1]BJS uses the first interview for bounding purposes only; it is not included in these data.

TABLE 2-1 Characteristics of Major Violence Against Women Datasets

Dataset	Sample	Frequency of Data Collection	Context of Survey	Has a Direct Question on Violence Against Women
Supplementary Homicide Reports (SHR)	Homicide incidents reported by police departments	Continuous	Criminal justice	Yes
National Crime Victimization Survey (NCVS)	National sample of households	Continuous	Criminal justice	Yes
National Incident-Based Reporting System (NIBRS)	Criminal incidents reported by law enforcement agencies	Continuous	Criminal justice	Yes
National Longitudinal Study of Adolescent Health—ADD Health (NLSAH)	National sample of adolescents, grades 7–12		Health	No
Monitoring the Future	National sample of 8th, 10th, and 12th graders	Continuous	Health	No
Pregnancy Risk Assessment Monitoring System (PRAMS)	Postpartum women from 32 states; oversampling of various racial/ ethnic groups and women who delivered low-birthweight children	Continuous	Health	Yes
National Youth Survey	National sample of youth		Criminal Justice	No

Use of Health or Social Services (by victim) Measured	Etiology[a]	Comorbid Factors[b] Can Be Assessed	Prevalence Data	Incidence Data	Chronicity Data
No	Yes	No	Yes	Yes	No
Health and some social	Potentially	Potentially	Potentially	Yes	Yes
No	No	No	No	Yes	No
Some health	Potentially	No	No	Yes	No
Some health and social	Potentially	Potentially	Potentially	Potentially	Potentially
No	No	No	No	Yes	No
No	Yes	Yes	Yes	Yes	Yes

Continued

TABLE 2-1 Continued

Dataset	Sample	Frequency of Data Collection	Context of Survey	Has a Direct Question on Violence Against Women
National Health and Social Life Survey (NHSLS)	National sample of general population, aged 18–59		Health	No
National College Health Risk Behavior Survey (NCHRBS)	National sample of undergraduate students		Health	No
National Ambulatory Medical Care Survey (NAMCS)	Physicians	Continuous	Health	No
National Hospital Ambulatory Medical Care Survey (NHAMCS)	National sample of patient record forms	Continuous	Health	No
National Hospital Discharge Survey (NHDS)	National sample of inpatient record forms for short-term hospital stays	Continuous	Health	No
National Health Interview Survey (NHIS)	National sample of households	Continuous	Health	No
National Survey of Family Growth (NSFG)	National sample of general population, aged 15–44	Continuous	Health	No
National Vital Statistics System (NVSS)	National sample of death certificates	Continuous	Health	No

Use of Health or Social Services (by victim) Measured	Etiology[a]	Comorbid Factors[b] Can Be Assessed	Prevalence Data	Incidence Data	Chronicity Data
Health	Yes	Yes	Yes	Yes	No
No	No	No	No	Yes	No
Health	No	Yes	No	No	No
Health	No	Yes	No	No	No
Health	No	Yes	No	No	No
Health and some social	Potentially	Yes	Potentially	Potentially	Potentially
Health	No	No	No	No	No
No	No	No	No	No	No

Continued

TABLE 2-1 Continued

Dataset	Sample	Frequency of Data Collection	Context of Survey	Has a Direct Question on Violence Against Women
National Morbidity Followback Survey (NMFS)	National sample of people who have died in a given year, with oversampling of African-Americans	Continuous	Health	No
National Electronic Injury Surveillance System (NEISS)	National sample of emergency room visits involving injuries	Continuous	Health	No
National Household Survey on Drug Abuse (NHSDA)	National sample of general population, aged 12 and up	Continuous	Health	No
National Violence Against Women Survey (NVAWS)	National sample of general population		Criminal justice	Yes
New Hampshire Youth at Risk	Sample of New Hampshire high school students		Health	Yes
National Surveys of Family Violence (NSFV)	National survey of families		Health	Yes
Youth Risk Behavior Surveillance System (YRBSS)	National sample of youth, grades 9–12	Continuous	Health	Yes
Behavioral Risk Factor Surveillance System (BRFSS)[c]	National sample of general population	Continuous	Health	Yes

effects on violence against women.

[a]Risk factors for intimate-partner violence.

[b]Other conditions that affect the magnitude of violence against women.

Use of Health or Social Services (by victim) Measured	Etiology[a]	Comorbid Factors[b] Can Be Assessed	Prevalence Data	Incidence Data	Chronicity Data
No	Yes	Yes	No	No	No
Health	No	No	No	No	No
No	Potentially	Yes	No	Yes	Yes
Health	Yes	Yes	Yes	Yes	Yes
No	Yes	Yes	No	No	No
Social	Yes	Yes	Yes	No	Yes
Health and social	Yes	No	Yes	Yes	Yes
No	Yes	Yes	Potentially	Potentially	No

[c]National data are derived from aggregating state statistics. States differ in their inclusion of questions on intimate-partner violence and in the types of questions asked.
NOTE: Where geocodes are available, linkages could be used to examine area spatial effects on violence against women.

lence perpetrated by both male and female members of a couple. Numerous research publications have resulted from the data collected, some estimating the prevalence of intimate-partner physical violence, and others examining associations between violence victimization and other topics (Gelles and Straus, 1988; Straus et al., 1988; Gelles, 1987; Straus, 1979). The completion rate for the first survey was 65 percent of the entire sample; 84 percent of eligible respondents completed the second survey (Straus and Gelles, 1986).

Despite the prominent role of the NSFV in research on partner violence, it has several well-known limitations. The CTS assess violence only in the context of a disagreement, and their earlier versions do not measure the severity of behaviors reported. Also, their original format did not assess a wide range of types of violence (including sexual violence). The new CTS2 includes emotionally abusive and sexually violent tactics and can be formatted so that the impact of a tactic is also measured. However, neither form of the CTS gathers information concerning whether the violence used was defensive in nature—a shortcoming of almost all current instruments employed in measuring intimate-partner violence. Because partner violence may best be conceptualized as a chronic condition that encompasses interrelated ongoing events, examining such violent behaviors out of context may miss important dimensions of the overall situation (Smith et al., 1999).

The National Violence Against Women Survey (NVAWS) was designed by Tjaden and Thoennes (1999) to remedy a limitation of the NCVS: because the NCVS is a general crime survey aimed at generating annual estimates of many types of crime, sample size constraints limit its usefulness as a source for better understanding historical and recent relational contexts likely to be associated with violence against women. Using a random-digit-dial household telephone survey, 8,000 women and 8,005 men aged 18 and older were sampled throughout the United States from November 1995 to May 1996. The interviews were completed by 72 percent of the women and 69 percent of the men sampled (Tjaden and Thoennes, 2000). The NVAWS employed a modified version of the CTS to collect data on physical assaults; data on sexual assaults and stalking, as well as injuries resulting from these victimization experiences, were also collected. This survey was unique among national surveys in its focus on respondents' lifetime histories of violence and its attention to gathering detailed information on perpetrators that could be linked across violent incidents. Despite these advantages, however, the NVAWS did not provide estimates of violent victimization that are comparable to those obtained by either the NCVS or the NSFV; the referent populations, some of the screening questions, and the quantification of series victimizations all differ. The NCVS focuses on assaults on respondents aged 12 and older, while the NVAWS focused on victimizations of respondents aged 18 and older. The NCVS also differs from the NVAWS in the approach used to count series victimizations.

The National Youth Survey is a nationally representative longitudinal survey of 1,725 persons who were aged 11–17 in 1976 when the study began and are now aged 37–43. The study has collected information on these individuals over time to assess their changing attitudes, beliefs, and behaviors with regard to deviance, exposure to delinquent peers, self-reported depression, delinquency, drug and alcohol use, victimization, pregnancy, abortion, use of mental health and outpatient services, violence by respondent and acquaintances, use of controlled drugs, and sexual activity. Data are available on the demographic and socioeconomic status of respondents, on parents and friends, and on neighborhood problems. The sample is 53 percent male and 47 percent female. The ethnicity of participants is comparable to that of the general population of the United States. The completion rate of eligible youth sampled was 73 percent in the initial wave of the survey; the completion rate of original respondents was 78 percent for the ninth wave in 1992 (Menard, 2002). This longitudinal survey reports on intimate-partner violence committed by both male and female respondents. Its estimates of lifetime prevalence are considerably higher than those derived from the surveys described above.

OTHER DATASETS

Supplementary Homicide Reports (SHR), part of the Federal Bureau of Investigation's Uniform Crime Reporting (UCR) program, is a major source of data on homicides (Bureau of Justice Statistics, 2002). Supplemental reports on homicide incidents have been voluntarily submitted monthly by local law enforcement agencies since 1976. These reports detail such information as age, race, and sex of victims and offenders, weapon use, circumstance of the crime, and the residential population and county and Metropolitan Statistical Area (MSA) codes of the reporting agency. SHR is particularly useful for research on intimate-partner homicide because it also collects data on the victim-offender relationship, categorized as intimate (spouse, ex-spouse, boyfriend, or girlfriend), other family, other acquaintance, or stranger. However, some limitations have been noted. First, supplemental reports are voluntary; about 91 percent of homicides reported in the UCR are included in SHR (Bureau of Justice Statistics, 2002). The actual incidence of homicides is underestimated compared with the National Vital Statistics System of the National Center for Health Statistics (Annest and Mercy, 1998). Also, ethnicity is determined by the observations of the reporting officer.

A number of other ongoing data collection efforts include questions on violence against women. Examples are the Behavioral Risk Factor Surveillance System, National Longitudinal Study of Adolescent Health, Pregnancy Risk Assessment Monitoring System, Youth Risk Behavior Surveillance System, National Health Interview Survey, and National Household Survey on Drug Abuse (for a more complete list, see Table 2-1). However, these surveys vary in the extent to which they systematically include measures of violence against women, gather data on the relationship between the victim and perpetrator, and address the situational context in which the violence occurs. The definitions and measures of violence against women used in these surveys also differ. Furthermore, these general population surveys rarely oversample racial minorities, and the data collection methods used (telephone and mail surveys) frequently preclude obtaining information on institutionalized and homeless women's experiences of violent victimization. Other one-time surveys have been conducted to measure various aspects of violence against women; these surveys are not described here (see, e.g., Fisher et al., 2000). There is also a handful of datasets from other countries that collect information on violence against women and could be expected to shed light on the problem in the United States. The following are examples of such datasets.

The Canadian Violence Against Women Survey examined the safety of women inside and outside the home. This survey, a one-time-only study based on a sample of households and conducted in 1993, served as a model for the NVAWS described above. Data elements collected in the Canadian survey included "perceptions of fear, sexual harassment, sexual violence, physical violence and threats by strangers, dates/boyfriends, other known men, husbands and common-law partners" (Statistics Canada, 1993). The target population for the survey was all Canadian women 18 years of age and over. Institutional populations and residents of the Yukon and Northwest Territories were excluded. The overall response rate was 54 percent. Canada also collects data annually on police-reported family violence.

The Dunedin Multidisciplinary Health and Development Study is a longitudinal investigation of a representative birth cohort of infants born between April 1, 1972, and March 31, 1973, in Dunedin, on New Zealand's South Island. The base sample was composed of 535 males and 502 females. The Dunedin birth cohort has been reassessed at 2-year intervals from ages 5 through 15 and at 3-year intervals between ages 15 and 21, with 97 percent of the living members of the age 3 base sample participating at age 21. The Dunedin data provide a unique opportunity for assessment of the developmental origins of partner violence that may have implications for understanding of the problem in the United States and elsewhere.

EXTENT AND NATURE OF VIOLENCE AGAINST WOMEN

Prevalence of Violence Against Women

Estimates of the prevalence of intimate-partner violence range widely, depending on the type of survey, the content of survey questions, and the sampling frame used (see Table 2-2). In nationally representative surveys in which women self-report physical abuse victimization by an intimate partner, past-year prevalence ranges from 0.43 percent of respondents to the NCVS reporting aggravated or simple assault to 11–12 percent of respondents to the NSFV reporting nonfatal physical abuse. In the five surveys that use the same measure—the CTS2—self-reports of intimate-partner physical abuse against women place past-year prevalence at 1.1–13.6 percent. In the four surveys that use the same measure plus comparable samples, the range is 1.1–9.1 percent for victimization in the past year.

Existing longitudinal studies place the past-year prevalence of intimate-partner physical abuse against women in the 20–50 percent range. Among all the surveys/studies of the prevalence of intimate-partner physical abuse victimization shown in Table 2-2, only the NCVS and the NVAWS report women's victimization as being higher than that of men; the others indicate that men report higher rates of severe and overall victimization. For the crime of rape, the NVAWS reports a prevalence 1.5 times higher than that reported in the NCVS. Only one of these surveys, the NCVS, is repeated at regular intervals, so that comparability among the various surveys—already compromised by differences in age range, sampling frame and sample sizes, length of recall period, and the manner in which questions are asked and violence is defined—is further diminished by differences in the reporting period. These kinds of conflicting prevalence rates make it impossible to develop credible estimates of trends over time or to determine the effectiveness of interventions.

Understanding Risk Factors

While existing datasets represent important strides in providing basic information about the overall scale and severity of violence against women, scholars are only beginning to learn about the risk factors for this particular type of violence. There is a long tradition of such research on other types of violence, such as violent delinquency. Risk factors for violence against women can reside in the individual victim, certain groups of women, characteristics of offenders, or social and spatial circumstances surrounding a violent event. However, as with risk factors identified in other criminology research, they cannot be used to predict a specific event

TABLE 2-2 Prevalence of Nonfatal Intimate-Partner Violence (IPV) Physical Abuse (Past Year)

Survey	Year	Sample	Measurement
National Prevalence Surveys			
National Surveys of Family Violence	1975	Households containing cohabiting (married or nonmarried) couple n = 2,143	Conflict Tactics Scale
	1985	Households containing cohabiting (married or nonmarried) couple n = 3,520	Conflict Tactics Scale, modified
National Alcohol and Family Violence Survey	1992	Married and cohabiting persons aged 18+ n = 1,970	Conflict Tactics Scale, modified
National Alcohol Survey	1995	Married and cohabiting couples n = 1,599 couples	Conflict Tactics Scale, modified
National Violence Against Women Survey	1995–1996	Persons aged 18+ n = 8,000 women, 8,000 men	Conflict Tactics Scale, modified
		Married and cohabiting persons aged 18+ n = 5,982 men, 5,655 women	Conflict Tactics Scale, modified
National Crime Victimization Survey	2001	Persons aged 12+ n = 79,950	
Longitudinal Studies			
Dunedin Multidisciplinary Health and Development Study	1993-1994	Study participants aged 21 who were in romantic relationships and their partners n = 360 couples	Physical abuse scale (CTS plus 4 additional items)
		Study participants aged 21 who were married or cohabiting n = 250	Conflict Tactics Scale
		Study participants age 21 who were married, cohabiting, or dating n = 861	Conflict Tactics Scale
National Youth Survey	1992	Study participants who were married or cohabiting n = 1,340	Conflict Tactics Scale

[a]Both partners reported the act occurred.
[b]Only respondent reported the act occurred.

% Reporting IPV Physical Abuse Victimization		
Female	Male	Total
12.1% overall, 3.8% severe	11.6% overall, 4.6% severe	16.0% overall, 6.1% severe
11.3% overall, 3.0% severe	12.1% overall, 4.4% severe	15.8% overall, 5.8% severe
9.1% overall, 1.9% severe	9.5% overall, 4.5% severe	
5.21%[a] to 13.61%[b]	6.22%[a] to 18.21%[b]	7.84%[a] to 21.48%[b]
1.3%	0.9%	
1.1%	0.6%	
0.43%	0.08%	0.26%
40.9%	47.4%	
38.8%	55.8%	
27.1% overall, 12.7% severe	34.1% overall, 21.2% severe	
20.2% any, 5.7% severe	27.9% any, 13.8% severe	

or to predict that a particular person will become a victim or an offender. They can often, however, indicate propensities for and patterns of risk by gender, race and ethnicity, and circumstances.

Gender

In general, overall victimization rates of women are low (compared with those of men or juveniles, for example)—an important reason for the almost total absence of research on this problem historically. However, the NCVS indicates that victimization by intimates accounts for 20 percent of violence experienced by women and 3 percent of that experienced by men (Rennison, 2003). Moreover, because women are most often victimized in "safe spaces" where no one witnesses the crime, they are more vulnerable to repeat attacks and are more likely to be severely injured or killed by intimate partners than by others. It is for these reasons that most research on the victimization of women has focused on intimate-partner violence (Bureau of Justice Statistics, 2000; Tjaden and Thoennes, 2000; National Research Council, 1996).

Interestingly, in nationally representative longitudinal studies in the United States and the above-described 21-year birth cohort study in New Zealand, women have reported higher levels of perpetration of intimate-partner violence than men, and men higher levels of victimization than women (Moffitt and Caspi, 1999). Some scholars have attributed this discrepancy to methodological problems in the CTS, which were used in these studies. Moreover, when serious violence (i.e., resulting in severe injury or death) is the focus, women do not report such higher levels of perpetration (Kruttschnitt, 2002). Moffitt and Caspi (1999) also note that male perpetrators are much more deviant (e.g., more likely to use illegal drugs or be chronically unemployed) than their female counterparts. Finally, it is intriguing to note that rates of violent victimization have been declining overall. However, violence against women for all crime types has been declining at lower rates than that against men (Bureau of Justice Statistics, 2000).

Race and Ethnicity

In a paper prepared for the workshop, Dugan and Apel (2002) use data from the NCVS over an 8-year period (January 1992 to June 2000) to model risk factors for all cases of nonlethal violent victimization of women. They note that until recently, researchers limited investigations of violence to African-American and white women, lumping groups such as Asian/Pacific Islanders and Native Americans into a generic "other" category or omitting them entirely (Dugan et al., 2000; Bureau of Justice Statistics, 2000; Greenfield et al., 1998).[2]

The usefulness of disaggregating female victims by race is underscored by the analysis of Dugan and Apel, who found that Native American women have considerably higher rates of victimization than other groups of women, they appear most likely to be victimized by someone they know, and their assailant is often using drugs or alcohol. Asian women have the highest proportion of incidents in public places and are more likely to be victimized by sober strangers or multiple offenders. White, African-American, and Hispanic teenage girls all have higher odds of victimization than young adult women, and those aged 60 or older display a significantly low risk. Having some college, but not 4 years, is positively related to violence for African-American and Hispanic women. Residential stability as measured by number of months living at the same location appears to lessen the risk for white and African-American women only.

Circumstances

Dugan and Apel (2002) found that the strongest risk factor for violent victimization of women is living in a household with one adult and children. This risk is greatest for Asian/Pacific Islander women. Controlling for other indicators of poverty, living in public housing is also a risk, especially for African-American and Hispanic women. Dugan and Apel (2002) conclude that living in the city, having more or younger children, or having low income appears to raise the risk of violence for all but Hispanic and Asian women. Moffitt and Caspi (1999) found that risk factors for female perpetrators of partner violence include disturbed family relationships, especially weak attachments, harsh discipline, and conflict between parents.

Although most research in this field reflects the belief that female victimization may be driven by some factors that differ from those affecting rates of male victimization, existing longitudinal studies point to risk factors that are similar to those for other kinds of criminal offending and victimization (Moffitt and Caspi, 1999; Straus and Gelles, 1992; Elliott et

---

[2]An important exception is the survey by Tjaden and Thoennes (2000), which describes differences in lifetime prevalence of violent victimization for Asian/Pacific Islander, Native American (including Alaskan Native), and mixed-race women (see also Rennison, 2001). Such analyses are, however, typically bivariate, leaving unanswered the question of which risk factors are of greater concern for any one group over the others.

al., 1986). Thus, an important research question is which risk factors specific to partner violence or other violence against women do not apply also to criminal offending or victimization in general. For example, most studies of homicide against women have been descriptive in nature and have focused on the murder of women by intimate male partners. More information about the characteristics of the killing of women in other circumstances would be helpful in understanding the lethal victimization of women in the context of homicide studies in general.

Health Consequences of Violence

It is widely recognized that violence against women, including intimate-partner violence, sexual assault, and rape, is associated with negative physical and mental health outcomes. Many studies have found a correlation between violence against women and emotional and physical health problems that go beyond the immediate effects of the abuse. Relationships have been found between previous physical abuse of women and stress-related physical health problems (Campbell et al., 2002b; Sutherland et al., 1998; Koss and Heslet, 1992), gynecological problems (Campbell et al., 2002b; Coker et al., 2000; Letourneau et al., 1999; Golding, 1996), and neurological injuries (Campbell et al., 2002b; Coker et al., 2000; Diaz-Olavarrieta et al., 1999). A recent meta-analysis revealed that women who experience domestic violence have elevated rates of insomnia, depression, post-traumatic stress disorder, panic disorder, and substance abuse—symptoms that can persist for years after the abuse ends (Golding, 1999).

One concern noted in *Understanding Violence Against Women* is that part of what is known about the health of abused women is provided by studies using samples drawn from women seeking medical care or from health plan populations. Such samples may not be representative of all victims: there may be differences in injury types, and uninsured women may not seek care. Hathaway et al. (2000) found that there was no difference between abused and nonabused women in rates of routine health care, although abused women were less likely to have health insurance. Lemon et al. (2002) report no differences in checkups and clinical breast examinations, but note that abused women are more likely to undergo Pap smear screening. However, findings of recent studies using population-based samples are largely consistent with findings of studies using clinic or health plan populations in showing that women who have been abused are more likely to report physical or emotional disabilities, smoking, unwanted pregnancy (Hathaway et al., 2000), high-risk alcohol use (Lemon et al., 2002), gynecologic problems (Plichta and Abraham, 1996), and mental health problems (Hathaway et al., 2000; Danielson et al., 1998).

In the Dunedin sample, 65 percent of women who had experienced severe abuse met criteria for one or more disorders listed in the Diagnostic and Statistical Manual of the American Psychiatric Association (DSM III-R). Abused women in this cohort were three times more likely than nonabused women to suffer a mental illness. Their disorders included depression, drug dependence, antisocial personality disorder, and schizophrenia (Moffitt and Caspi, 1999).

An important concern remains with regard to establishing causality. Most studies focus on correlates of violence, failing to establish the temporal sequence of events and leaving the pathways between abuse and health outcomes unspecified. Many victims of intimate-partner violence have reported problems, such as unemployment, lack of transportation, substandard housing, and financial difficulties, that may predispose women to poor health outcomes (Browne et al., 1999; Eby, 1996; Sullivan et al., 1992). One population-based study, by Sutherland et al. (2001), addressed this problem by investigating whether intimate-partner violence has a significant effect on women's health beyond that which can be explained by poverty. Both income and physical abuse contributed to women's rates of physical health symptoms, and abuse contributed to the variance in physical health beyond that predicted by income level alone. Additional research is needed to further explain the direct and indirect causes of health problems experienced by victims of abuse.

Risk of Injury and Death

Dugan and Apel (2002) measured the likelihood of injury in all types of violent crimes against women. They found that crimes involving physical contact with known persons and the presence of a weapon were predictors of severe injury. According to the NVAWS, 36 percent of women who had been raped since age 18 and 42 percent of women who had been physically assaulted since age 18 reported that they had been injured during their most recent victimization. However, most of the injuries were relatively minor (scratches, bruises, welts), while more serious injuries (broken bones, dislocated joints, concussions, lacerations, bullet wounds) were sustained by relatively few of the victims (Tjaden and Thoennes, 2000). In a study by the RAND Corporation, intimate-partner violence was found to be one of the most common causes of injury in women (Rand, 1997).

When survivors of serious injury are compared with those who were killed, findings suggest that women who are harmed by their husbands, as opposed to a live-in boyfriend or acquaintance, are overrepresented as victims of homicide (Dugan and Apel, 2002). The Dunedin study found that men who severely injured their partners demonstrated extreme levels of deviance as characterized by polydrug use, antisocial personality disorder, chronic unemployment, and violent acts against persons outside the family (Moffitt and Caspi, 1999). In preliminary findings from her study of women killed by their intimate partners, Campbell (2002) found the most important pre-incident demographic risk factor in predicting lethality in abusive relationships to be perpetrator unemployment.

Dawson (2002) describes a recent framework that has been applied to understanding declines in intimate-partner homicide (see also Dugan et al., 1999, 2000). The "exposure reduction" framework highlights key social changes that may have contributed to the decline in intimate-partner homicide in recent decades. These include changes in the nature of intimate relationships—fewer and/or delayed marriages and more divorce; improved socioeconomic status of women, including increasing gender equality; and the increased availability of domestic violence resources, including legal and social services (e.g., domestic violence courts, shelters). Considering that intimate-partner homicide is often preceded by a history of intimate-partner violence, the exposure reduction framework holds that the impact of social changes that help abused women exit violent relationships or prevent women from entering such relationships may also reduce the rate of intimate lethal victimization. Further research is needed on the potential of this framework for increasing understanding of murders and assaults of women. If we are to be able to prevent such crimes, moreover, longitudinal research in the United States is needed to determine which risk factors (if any), for which groups of women, are truly unique to lethal events or outcomes involving severe injury. The committee recommends that work be initiated to examine the feasibility and cost-effectiveness of successfully conducting such longitudinal studies.

METHODOLOGICAL ISSUES

Improving Measurement

As noted above, many federally and some privately sponsored data collections include information on violence against women. As noted earlier, in 1998, NIJ and CDC sponsored a conference on improving research on violence against women. The matrix produced at that conference (the basis for Table 2-1) categorizes the existing datasets relevant to this research according to the following characteristics:

• Whether the survey was a one-time only study or continuous. Continuous was defined as conducted at regular intervals (e.g., every 6 months in the case of the NCVS, annually in the case of the Youth Risk Behavior Survey) and expected to be conducted (repeated) in the future.

• Whether the survey was precise (generally defined as designed to minimize standard measurement errors).

• Whether a supplement or follow-back could be undertaken to better estimate violence against women.

• Whether the survey was a health or criminal justice survey.

• Whether there was a social service utilization measure for violence against women.

• Whether risk factors for violence against women could be estimated from the survey.

Despite the variations in the quality of the various surveys listed in Table 2-1, creating linkages among existing survey data would provide important additional resources for scholars interested in the contexts and outcomes of violent victimization. Generally, such linkages will not be possible across individuals in the different datasets but may be possible across common geographic areas, for example, states or cities. In addition, linkages between national-level surveys can be developed that relate differing characteristics of events to one another. A good example is the research on the outcomes of violent victimization based on the merging of data from the SHR with NCVS data (see Felson and Messner, 1996; Kleck and McElrath, 1991). If the NCVS could be linked to data from the National Health Interview Survey, information could be obtained on health-related outcomes of violent injuries. Research is needed on the feasibility of linking different datasets and on how to validate survey data with data on clinical, legal, and social outcomes. An important aspect of this linking process will be developing a framework for standard definitions.

To advance understanding of violence against women, the constructs researchers use must be valid and reliable across different social settings, samples, and measurement conditions. Currently, the behaviors used to measure or operationalize "violence" or abuse are wide-ranging, and this seriously compromises our understanding of the prevalence and distribution of violence against women. For example, even where the same measures and comparable samples are used, prevalence estimates differ by a factor of 2 (see Moffitt and Caspi, 1999). Part of the problem is a lack of information on the amount of harm or the nature of an injury resulting from a violent act. As Johnson (1995) demonstrates, research that uses the CTS and does not tap the consequences of various violent tactics comes to a very different conclusion about the prevalence of violent victimization among men and women than would be derived from agency or official data. Although much of Johnson's argument revolves around sampling issues rather than measurement issues, there is no question that differences in what is counted as a violent act (e.g., pushed or shoved versus broken bones) affect how many women and men are classified as victims of intimate-partner violence. These discrepancies in findings raise a central question: What elements should be included in the definition of violence, or what kinds of behaviors should be considered violent? Cook (2000) documents at least 29 different measurement instruments used in research on violence against women. These measures vary not only in the types, levels, and degrees of coercion they measure, but also in the severity of the acts they include. Rigorous inquiry into violence against women is precluded when scholars fail to distinguish among what constitutes an act of violence, abuse, or battering.

The NSFV suggests that abuse has a normative criterion but uses the terms "abuse," "assault," and "violence" relatively interchangeably, differentiating only between what are termed "minor" and "severe" violent acts based on the potential risk of injury (Straus and Gelles, 1992:75–85). These terms fail to distinguish among physical violence, physical aggression, and psychological abuse. This lack of conceptual and operational clarity is particularly problematic when attempts are made to compare survey findings with data on clinical populations, among whom abuse may be determined by specific medical criteria. It is also problematic considering that what constitutes being victimized and what constitutes offending may be culturally determined. If we want to be able to determine whether critical aspects of abusive and violent behaviors against women (e.g., their prevalence, incidence, and distribution) differ from those of other kinds of violent behavior, we need to employ consistent definitions and measures.

This distinction between nominal and operational definitions applies not just to questions of how violence or abuse is measured, but also to questions of how different research settings introduce measurement problems. Violence may be operationalized differently in clinical, legal, and research settings or, as occurred in the redesign of the NCVS in 1992, even within the same setting over different periods of time.

Causes, correlates, and epidemiological and survey estimates of violence may all be sensitive to the conceptual and operational clarity of definitions. Far more than half of violent crimes against women remain unredressed, in large part because they are unknown to criminal justice authorities. Scholars have developed some important methods for assessing this so-called "dark figure of crime," but a large proportion of violent crimes perpetrated between intimates and family members are still unreported.

Improving Research

The committee recommends more research to examine the situational contexts and dynamic interactions that lead to violence against women. Research on violent events complements studies of the individual propensities of victims or offenders, and focuses instead on the *occurrence* of violence, identifying the specific conditions that channel individual motivation and predispositions into violent actions. This approach addresses the social or psychological pathways that bring individuals to specific violent events and the transactions or decisions that comprise the onset, course, conclusion, and aftermath of the event.

Recent studies on interpersonal violence among strangers illustrate the confluence of motivation, perceptions of risk and opportunity, and the social control attributes of the setting that shapes the decision to participate in a violent event, as well as its outcome (Wilkinson and Fagan, 2001). Other research shows that violence against women serves specific functions for assailants, and that those functions may covary with the type of assault. Tedeschi and Felson (1994) hypothesize that all violence is related to one or more of the following three goals: compliance, identity, and justice. To understand the catalyst for a violent event among intimates, researchers must examine the social construction and discourse on male–female relationships, perceived imbalances in power, control dynamics, identity threats, relationship problems, and communication patterns . It is important to recognize that "when violence occurs it is not an isolated event in peoples' lives, but is embedded firmly in the process of interpersonal communication which people use to regulate their lives" . Research on the "sparks," motivations, interaction patterns, and decision making associated with violent events can identify leverage points for reducing the threat of violence or averting it entirely.

Some violent events against female victims are stranger assaults, and understanding the situational and structural contexts of those events provides another window on social factors that elevate risks beyond those attributable to individual offenders or victims. While women's victimization results from various forms of violence, there are commonalities across those events that can be examined to provide a differentiated understanding of the unique and shared risks involved. The following are some examples of research on situational contexts and violent interactions:

• *Research on the processes of victim selection*—Stranger assaults may appear at first glance to be random occurrences, but there are processes of victim selection that can be studied to identify attributes of individuals, settings, and social interactions that may motivate victim selection.

- *Research on location selection*—The selection of locations for assaults against women may reflect a rational decision-making process that can be modified to reduce risk and prevent physical or sexual assault.
- *Research on victim–offender interaction patterns*—Studies of the patterns of social interaction in stranger violence have generated robust theories of violent interaction that can be extended to the unique circumstances of gender-related assaults. Studies of these interaction patterns in domestic violence show how personality factors interact with situational contexts to launch interaction dynamics that end in assaults by male intimate partners against women (see Jacobson and Gottman, 1998; Wilkinson and Hamerschlag, 2002; Wilkinson and Fagan, 2001). Replications and extensions of this research should encompass a more diverse set of relationships and different types of assault. These studies should examine and decompose the stages of violent events—from arousal to aggression—to identify behavioral scripts or cognitive frames that are amenable to intervention or prevention efforts.

Several datasets currently available can be examined to begin the process of theory construction. Research designs using survey methods, event history research with samples of individuals, and laboratory experiments can begin to generate the empirical data that will produce a more refined and productive knowledge base from which prevention efforts can be launched.

CONCLUSION

Although progress has been made in the effort to measure and understand the nature of violence against women, a more coordinated research strategy would help remedy the measurement problems that remain. The committee recommends that an effort be made to investigate how to link different datasets and how to link information from these datasets with findings from clinical research to provide more information on the risks of, responses to, and consequences of violence against women and the impact of interventions. Such an effort should include the formulation of a framework for developing standard definitions to overcome the lack of conceptual and operational clarity, as well as other problems involved in measuring violence against women, especially differences in sample selection among studies. In addition, more attention should be devoted to developing event-based measures of violence against women.

3

Social Ecological Risks of Violence Against Women

Research on violence against women has focused primarily on individual characteristics of victims or offenders or on event-level or situational characteristics of assaults and other forms of violence. For many years, it was widely thought that violence against women was "classless"; that is, women were victimized at high rates regardless of their socioeconomic status or the neighborhood in which they lived (Straus et al., 1980). Findings of research in the 1970s indicated that the spatial dimensions of violence against women were unimportant since intimate-partner violence and rape were both well distributed by race and social class.

This neglect of social context in research on violence against women is surprising given the current widespread recognition of the significance of community characteristics and neighborhood effects for violence generally (Fagan, 1993), for the actual socioeconomic distribution of both victimization and offending behavior by women (Rennison and Welchans, 2000), and for other related social problems. Indeed, recent research provides evidence for community effects on violence and social problems that may be gender-specific, including child abuse (Coulton et al., 1995; Coulton and Padney, 1992; Zuravin, 1989; Garbarino and Sherman, 1980), teenage pregnancy (Sullivan, 1993, 1989), the prevalence of marital versus cohabiting living arrangements (Tucker and Mitchell-Kernan, 1995; Sullivan, 1993), and the prevalence of female-headed households (Stokes and Chevan, 1996; Tucker and Mitchell-Kernan, 1995). The remainder of this chapter reviews what research tells us about the importance of social context for both intimate-partner violence and sexual assault by strangers, and describes research and data needs in this important area of study.

A number of recent studies have shown that rates of violence against women vary across such social areas as census tracts and neighborhoods (Miles-Doan, 1998). Moreover, the geographic distribution of violent victimization of women overlaps to a large degree with that of male victimization (Fagan et al., 2002). This finding is perhaps easier to understand once we confront the fact that most violence against both men and women is perpetrated by men (Tjaden and Thoennes, 2000).

Some studies have shown that violent victimization of women, and particularly the risk of injury or fatality, is concentrated among poor, non-white populations. Prevalence estimates for stranger-perpetrated violence may be conservative for the neighborhoods in which these women live, and this exposure to violence by strangers also may contribute to factors that characterize violent offending by women (Baskin and Sommers, 1998). Even intimate-partner violence appears to be susceptible to neighborhood effects. Block and Christakos (1995) found that the hardening, or general violence, of the inner city had an impact on female victimization by partners.

Other research has shown that the effects of criminal legal sanctions for domestic violence covary with neighborhood context (Benson et al., 2003; Wooldredge and Thistlethwaite, 2002) or that the availability of services leads to declines in intimate-partner homicide (Dugan et al., 2000; Browne and Williams, 1989). Moreover, just as individuals change over time in their rates of violent offending or victimization, so, too, do violence rates in cities and neighborhoods (Taylor and Covington, 1988). For example, Medina (2002a) discusses the idea that neighborhoods have a natural history of violence, with rates increasing and decreasing over time in relation to changes in both social structural factors and other social problems, such as drug or violence epidemics.

These simple empirical facts, when framed in the context of theories of the risk of community-level violence, invite closer examination of the social ecological contexts of violence against women. The studies described above have extended advances in theory and research on communities and crime to the study of violence against women. These studies have applied social structural theories and dynamic theories of social organization and social control to explain variation across neighborhoods or cities in rates of violence against women. Even with this knowledge, however, virtually no research has compared social or neighborhood risks of violence for female and male victims. Nor has research examined the links between the patterns of victimization of women and men in a broader analysis of the spatial ecology of violence.

INTIMATE-PARTNER VIOLENCE

In a paper prepared for the workshop, Medina (2002b) observes that attempts to explain concentrations of violence against women using measures of gender inequality point instead to the relevance of other community characteristics. In 1927, Mowrer suggested that spatial patterns of marital conflict, particularly divorce and desertion, can be explained within a social disorganization framework. Some authors have argued that the mechanisms at play are those emphasized by contemporary versions of social disorganization theory.

Fagan (1993) offers the most developed interpretation of the geography of intimate-partner violence consistent with this framework (see also Williams and Hawkins, 1992, 1989a, 1989b). For Fagan, the relevant dimensions of community for understanding spouse assault include the level of social control within the community, the social networks within which people and couples are embedded, and the community's social capital. The concentration of social structural deficits in urban areas weakens both informal and formal social controls on spouse assault.

The significance of social networks for spouse assault is illustrated by researchers' understanding of both the risk factors involved and the importance of victims' ability to invoke informal social controls. Social isolation is a risk factor for domestic violence (Stets, 1991; Thompson et al., 2000), but the effects of social isolation also increase the risks of partner violence at the community level. Growing residential segregation and isolation of residents from the social and economic institutions that represent mainstream society weaken the influence of the larger society on interpersonal behaviors, particularly among the minority groups segregated in inner-city areas. The absence of patterns of husband-wife interaction more commonly transmitted by working families embedded in stable kinship or friendship networks facilitates the transmission and reification of more-violent norms (Massey and Denton, 1993).

SEXUAL ASSAULT BY STRANGERS

Whereas the study of the spatial dynamics of physical violence against women by their intimate partners has been dominated by a focus on the "neighborhood" and structural factors, the study of stranger rape has been dominated by the "place" and opportunity research tradition. Medina (2002b) found an extensive body of research examining the spatial predatory patterns of the search for victims in which serial rapists engage. These crimes are more likely to be reported than the much more common nonstranger sexual assaults. Serial rapists, moreover, have a tendency to use the same space repeatedly (LeBeau, 1987), to the point where they influence the definition of those areas with the highest incidence of rape (LeBeau, 1985).

This research documents the distance from the rapist's home to the points where victims are located and raped (Myers et al., 1998; Warren et al., 1998; Kocsis and Irwin, 1997; LeBeau, 1992, 1979; Costanzo et al., 1986; Rand, 1984). Medina (2002b) suggests that by inverting the findings of this research, one can deduce the probable residence of an offender from information about the known crime locations, their geographic connections, and their characteristics. Indeed, police departments in several countries are using computerized geographic profiling in their investigations of serial sexual assaults with an acceptable degree of success (Rossmo, 1995). This intervention may not have applicability, however, to the majority of sexual assaults, which, according to Tjaden and Thoennes (2000), are perpetrated by intimate partners.

RESEARCH NEEDS

The findings and questions resulting from recent research on community effects suggest first steps toward integrating theory and research on the social ecological characteristics of violence and on the epidemiology of violence against women. The research agenda that emerges from a consideration of this work addresses a series of important scientific questions, as detailed below.

Social and Spatial Epidemiology of Violence

Research is needed to estimate the extent of variation in violence against women across census tracts or small neighborhoods, police precincts or districts, or other theoretically meaningful social area aggregations. For example, it may be found that rates of violence against women vary at the census tract or neighborhood level, but that these differences are masked at higher units of aggregation, such as planning districts comprising several tracts. Such research may also reveal that there are differences in area risks for different forms of violence against women. A corollary question is whether these differences persist over time, or whether there are variations in the stability of violence rates for different area units or different types of victimization. That is, an important research question is whether life history and ethnographic methods can be applied to neighborhoods or other small social areas to identify factors that elevate or attenuate rates of violence against women and if so, which forms of violence are thus affected. Research designs should specify which areal units are important for which theoretical perspectives, what data are available at those levels, and whether critical data are lacking.

A related question is the interdependence of violence against women and violence against men in the same social areas. Research should explore this question by estimating the covariance of the two violence rates over time at different units of spatial aggregation. For example, it is important to know whether increases in rates of violence against men elevate the risks of violence against women over time. To determine whether correspondence in these rates is spurious, it is important to construct better ecology models that take gender into account.

Social Area Risks of Violence Against Women

Research is needed to determine which features of area composition influence rates and types of violence against women. As suggested above, understanding the social structural, social organizational, and social control capacities of neighborhoods is critical to explaining differences in rates of violence against women. A related question is whether changes in these social area features predict changes in violence rates over time. For example, research should explore whether changes in marriage rates or wages for women predict changes in rates of violence against women. Similarly, research should examine whether an increase in men's unemployment rate or educational attainment is associated with an increase in violence against women (Macmillan and Gartner, 1999). Often researchers studying neighborhood ecology must deal with aggregation bias that may confound individual effects with effects of neighborhood context and therefore fail to detect true ecological effects. This problem can be minimized by using independent measures of individual status (e.g., employment, education) and neighborhood context (Simcha-Fagan and Schwartz, 1986; Sampson et al., 1997).

An important task for this research is to estimate whether there are gender-specific dimensions of a neighborhood that elevate violence risks for women beyond the overall risks of violence in that area. Thus, for example, research should test whether sex ratios, women's participation in labor markets, wage differentials, or other gender-specific social structural features of neighborhoods are associated with particular risks of violence against women. A further question is whether these gender-specific area risks vary for different forms of victimization. Both epidemiologically and theoretically, research should formulate separate models for violence against women and against men, and then explicitly test their interdependence.

Distribution of Services

One dimension of social ecology is access to different types of services. The availability of services (e.g., shelters, counseling) has been linked to variation in rates of intimate-partner homicides against women

(Browne and Williams, 1989; Dugan et al., 2000), but only in state- or city-level analyses. Whether access to local services, and at what distance from event locations, can affect localized rates of intimate-partner violence is a critical research question with important implications for the planning and location of preventive services. Research should examine, for example, the relationship between violence "hot spots" and service locations to assess distances that are barriers to the prevention or deterrence of intimate-partner violence. Research on the locations of other services, including counseling centers and medical services, also should examine this relationship. Research should consider whether access to gender-specific services or general violence prevention services, and at what distance from event locations, may make a difference in the occurrence of victimization.

Social Area Effects on Sanctions and Services

Social ecological factors may affect not only rates of violence, but also the efficacy of legal sanctions and social interventions. For example, the effects of arrest on the recurrence of intimate-partner violence vary with the social position of both victim and offender (Sherman and Smith, 1992; Maxwell et al., 2001). But the clustering of persons of similar social positions in neighborhoods or other homogeneous social areas suggests that areas themselves may influence aggregate rates of compliance with legal sanctions (see, for example, Mears et al., 2001). Additionally, research has shown that dynamic processes of social control affect violence rates in neighborhoods (Dekeseredy et al., 2003; Sampson and Bartusch, 1998; Sampson et al., 1997), as well as rates of intimate-partner violence (Browning, in press).

Despite these advances in knowledge, however, research is needed to examine the covariation of individual and social area factors in the responses of both victims and offenders to legal sanctions or social interventions for violence against women. Sanctions may have a deterrent effect in neighborhoods where the social and legal costs of offending are high to perpetrators, but may have the opposite effect in areas where high rates of poverty or social exclusion mitigate both the social costs of offending and the punishment costs of sanctions. Research on this topic should examine not only small areas (such as neighborhoods), but also police districts and other areas where law enforcement strategies are implemented and managed. Research is needed as well on area effects on different forms of violence against women.

DATA NEEDS

To create a data infrastructure that can be used to test the above research questions, modifications will be needed in the sampling strategies employed in survey research and epidemiological studies so that social ecological factors can be incorporated. Stratified sampling designs in survey and epidemiological research should include samples of social areas, as well as of individuals within areas. The selection of social areas should reflect the theoretical question at hand. Studies of the effects of policing, for example, might include both police districts and social neighborhoods as ecological sampling units.

The types of data collected on social areas also should reflect theoretical questions. Studies of informal social control, for example, should include survey data from individuals who can report on the social organization and dynamic processes of social control within an area (for an example, see Sampson et al., 1997). To avoid aggregation biases, these samples should be independent of the samples of individuals from whom epidemiological data on the incidence of violent victimization are collected. To obtain accurate estimates of the covarying influences of individual and area characteristics, the methods of data analysis employed must estimate multilevel effects and avoid the problems of clustering of individual and neighborhood risks (i.e., endogeneity) that often occur in hierarchical studies of violent victimization.

The advances in crime mapping methods discussed above can be extended to the study of violent victimization of women. Administrative records from law enforcement and other criminal justice or social service agencies can be modified to include addressable data for events, victims, and offenders. Possible sources of information on victimization of women might also include probability samples on health and victimization and certain public health and vital statistics records (e.g., those who seek treatment, those who are murdered or commit suicide). The integration of public health and criminal justice records, if feasible, might provide more robust estimates of the prevalence of violence against women at various levels of aggregation that would avoid the biases of the respective systems.

4

Prevention and Deterrence[1]

This chapter reviews research on prevention and deterrence efforts undertaken at various levels of government and by private organizations to reduce violence against women. It also identifies research needed to better understand what does and does not work in preventing and deterring these violent behaviors.

AN EPIDEMIOLOGICAL MODEL

Public health models can be applied to the problem of violence against women using the traditional framework of primary, secondary, and tertiary prevention. Primary prevention effects a change in risk factors. Its purpose is to prevent disease or injury, which in the case of violence against women means preventing the assault or abusive behavior from happening in the first place through, for example, the strengthening of protective factors. Secondary prevention is early identification. Its purpose is to reduce the risk of death or disability, for example, through screening and follow-up care. Tertiary prevention is a response to an event, such as a domestic violence assault. Its purpose from a public health point of view is to extend life after the event; an example in the case of

---

[1]Prevention involves programs and services available to victims and offenders that aim to decrease the number of new cases of assault or abusive behavior, reduce the risk of death or disability from violence, and extend life after a violent event; deterrence involves the use of sanctions to prevent offenders from using violence.

violence against women is psychological counseling to deal with the trauma of abuse.

Most of the funding available for the prevention of intimate-partner violence and sexual assault is spent on tertiary prevention, or treatment. In public health, tertiary prevention is designed to effect major behavior changes in individuals. A public health prevention research agenda would seek to learn enough about risk factors to evaluate interventions starting in childhood and adolescence, and identify and target social norms condoning violence.

Primary Prevention

In primary prevention, strategies and programs should be based on plausible and stable theories or causes and should be rigorously evaluated. Current primary prevention strategies focusing on the first occurrence of violence include offering school-based training in conflict resolution, educating the public about healthy relationships, providing early sex education, limiting children's exposure to sexually violent and aggressive media images, targeting specific interventions for children witnessing partner violence, and integrating training in parenting skills into school health curricula. There has been no evaluation of the effectiveness of most of these strategies in reducing violence; experimental studies are needed for this purpose.

Secondary Prevention

One objective of secondary prevention of violence against women is moderating the level of violence. Among suggested strategies for this purpose in the case of intimate-partner violence are the use of screening mechanisms for abuse, including psychological abuse, in health care and social service settings and training of health care workers to identify physical and sexual violence. Another objective of secondary prevention is to moderate or eliminate exposure to the violence, for example, by providing protective orders and relocation for victims. A third objective is to modify the relevant characteristics of the hazard through such services as supportive counseling and crisis hot lines, aimed at persons at risk of becoming offenders to reduce aggression. Finally, secondary prevention can be aimed at making victims more resistant to damage, through such efforts as counseling, self-defense classes, and strengthening of community mental health services for victims and their families. Research is still needed in many of these areas, as discussed later in the chapter.

Tertiary Prevention

The first objective of tertiary prevention is to counter the damage done by an assault. Means of accomplishing this objective include the criminal justice response, as well as medical, legal, and advocacy services to victims. Batterer education programs might also be included in this category. Evaluating the effectiveness of these strategies requires information from both victims and abusers. It is important to note that coordinated community responses to violence against women should be expanded to treat the psychological impact of the violence and should ensure that victims have access to the services they need.

OTHER RESEARCH ON PREVENTION

Specific information about violent crimes—including victim, offender, and situation or place (see Chapter 3)—is critical to the design of appropriate research programs that can support prevention efforts (Block, 2002). Reliance on aggregate statistics to understand intimate-partner homicide has been shown to mask important differences and lead to ineffective targeting of services. Specific information—such as marital status, age, and prior victimization experience, which have been shown to be risk factors—is important for prioritizing prevention efforts and targeting them to specific groups (Bureau of Justice Statistics, 2002).

The design of projects targeting batterers and potential batterers must be sensitive to different cultural backgrounds, including the importance assigned to having an intact family in a given culture, and to different kinds of family situations and arrangements. It is also important to look at patterns of violent behavior and the risk of violence over the life span of both offenders and their victims in different settings (see also Chapter 3). One example of an important contextual issue is the role of guardians or potential guardians in establishing safety for victims. Potential guardians—friends, neighbors, faith communities, the health community, and the criminal justice community—often do not know what to do when someone asks for help. Very few women talk to counselors—only about 15 percent according to Block (2002)—and those that do so turn first to guardians because they are the gatekeepers. Yet no evaluative research has been done on what gatekeepers and guardians need to know for successful interventions, and little research exists on what defines a safe place.

Changing Attitudes, Beliefs, and Behaviors
Among At-Risk Populations

In their review of efforts to prevent violence against women, Maxwell and Post (2002) note that since the mid-1980s, colleges and universities across the United States have begun to offer educational programs that address sexual violence (see also Roark, 1987). This effort was enhanced in the early 1990s with the passage of two federal laws providing financial resources to rape crisis centers, nonprofit entities, and schools to support educational programs designed to increase awareness and help prevent sexual assault, intimate-partner violence, and sexual harassment.

Unfortunately, the substantial variation among education intervention models has led to little cumulative or synthesized knowledge about effective methods of delivering such education and offered limited understanding of both its proximal and distal preventive effects (Breitenbecher, 2000; McCall, 1993). Maxwell and Post (2002) believe this may be because preventive education programs have been designed to provide a complete package of treatments to cover all possible causes of violence against women (Schewe and O'Donohue, 1993:668). Nevertheless, while assessing the research on these interventions, Maxwell and Post note several themes:

- The nature and quality of the evaluation designs varied significantly. Evaluations ranged, for example, from a pre- and post-test design involving a single treatment group (see Ellis et al., 1992) to more rigorous methods, such as a study that used a Solomon four-group design (see Fonow et al., 1992).
- Only weak associations were found between sexual assault–related attitudes and behavior. Two of the three studies measuring actual behavior (e.g., dating behavior) found that the programs were not effective in reducing the incidence of victimization (Breitenbecher, 2000).
- Except for a handful of evaluations, most studies did not provide long-term follow-up by testing or retesting their subjects on either attitude or behavior.
- Additional research suggests that the growth of these prevention programs has not had a contagious effect on the targeted population. Woods and Bower (2001) note that students in 2001 answered questions about date rape very similarly to those in the early 1980s and 1990s.

Changing the Opportunities for Violence Through "Target Hardening"

Maxwell and Post (2002) note that during the 1990s, theoretical work was done on why victims, offenders, and crime are environmentally concentrated (see, e.g., Eck and Weisburd, 1995; Miethe, 1994; Felson, 1987; Garofalo, 1987). Scholars investigating violence against women demonstrated that sexual assault (LeBeau, 1994; Schewe and O'Donohue, 1993; Sanday, 1981) and intimate-partner violence (Lemon, 1996; Campbell, 1992) are not equally distributed spatially or temporally (see, e.g., Kayitsinga and Maxwell, 2000; Baron and Straus, 1989).

Thus it has been argued that environmental strategies designed to make crime more difficult to commit can facilitate prevention. Such strategies include, for example, "target hardening" and the concentration of limited law enforcement resources. According to Schewe and O'Donohue (1993), the prevention technique most often used involves activities self-initiated by women and informed by the temporal and spatial patterns of rape to reduce opportunities for an assault. A majority of the women in the study, regardless of their expressed fear of rape, reported taking steps to reduce the risk of rape, such as carrying keys in their hand. More recently, sexual assault prevention programs and the literature have also emphasized situational precautions a woman can take to prevent the introduction of a "date rape" drug into her drink without her knowledge. From the public health perspective of primary prevention, these types of efforts are about strengthening the woman's ability to resist environmental stressors (Bloom, 1981).

In addition to such self-initiated steps taken by women, both public and private agencies have undertaken efforts to reduce the opportunities for rape. Universities, police departments, private property managers (Shenkel, 1989), and other public agencies have, for example, installed emergency phones, increased lighting, tightened security in residence halls, provided escort services, and increased the number of police in certain areas. Congress also acknowledged the importance of this prevention model by including two sections in the Violence Against Women Act of 1994 that authorized spending $25 million for capital improvement projects to increase safety in urban parks, recreation areas, and public transportation areas. Unfortunately, in their review, Maxwell and Post (2002) could find no published evaluation of efforts to prevent violence against women by reducing opportunities.

Self-Defense Models

Self-defense techniques—defined as "psychological, verbal, and physical resistance in dangerous situations when they arise" (Rozee and Koss, 2002:12)—are taught in programs that typically focus on increasing women's physical self-defense skills and their use of physical and psychological strategies to set boundaries and boost self-esteem (Thompson, 1991). Indeed, self-defense techniques may be among the most widely promoted tools for preventing violence against women. Maxwell and Post (2002) found more than 20,000 websites that discussed, promoted, or sold goods and services for women's self-defense.

An overabundance of empirical research on outcomes of self-defense measures taken by women is noted in *Understanding Violence Against Women*. Ullman's (1997) review of self-defense studies includes 31 published studies of situational and behavioral factors related to rape avoidance. Maxwell and Post's (2002) assessment of these studies is similar to that of other reviewers: there is sufficient indication that women who resist a rape attempt are more likely to thwart the attack and not incur more serious injuries (Rozee and Koss, 2002; National Research Council, 1996). No systematic assessments of whether self-defense programs increase the effectiveness of self-defense measures over what women can achieve without such training were found, however.

Evaluation of Preventive Programs

Schematic models help in visualizing all of the elements involved in an act of violence and the many possible points of intervention. Consider a simple three-part model, for example, based on the assumption that violence causes injuries because it involves a transfer of energy from perpetrator to victim via a weapon: victim-weapon-perpetrator. This simple model suggests two points of intervention—between perpetrator and weapon and between weapon and victim. Laws controlling access to guns are an example of interventions in the former category, while safe houses for battered women are among interventions in the latter. Such simple models can be elaborated more fully as research helps us understand what factors are involved at each point in the process. Knowledge of the situation in which perpetrator and victim are likely to find themselves is an example of the kind of information that can inform the design and implementation of interventions that are likely to be effective.

Determining whether a specific intervention works depends on evaluation that assesses the process of program implementation as well as final outcomes. Formative evaluation that yields a rich description of the process of intervention is helpful to the field because it provides information about possible interactions. Regardless of whether the final outcome proves statistically significant, such evaluation can aid in formulating new hypotheses and better-informed plans for intervention.

Assessments of program outcomes that specify and operationalize desired outcomes are critical to scientific research and helpful to program designers in determining whether a program can achieve the desired goals. As the principle of evidence-based practice gains currency, however, the demand for evaluation studies that meet high standards for both design and implementation is likely to grow. The National Task Force on Community Preventive Services, like other groups that assess the evidence base for practice, uses an algorithm to assess the quality of published studies and reports. A crucial factor for meeting such standards is the use of comparison groups and substantial follow-up. Both of these requirements raise the level of scientific expertise needed for the design of an intervention, as well as its cost. Nonetheless, it has become apparent from the work of the National Task Force on Community Preventive Services and other evidence-based review groups that the systematic review of a body of literature makes an important contribution to determining what works. The Centers for Disease Control and Prevention (CDC) has begun to use such information both to encourage the use of effective programs and to promote research in areas in which there is insufficient evidence to make decisions about specific interventions. This judicious use of resources is likely to speed the development and widespread implementation of effective practice.

Legal Reforms

Although sanctions against wife abuse have historically been part of many state criminal codes, criminal justice institutions have reacted toward violence against women with ambivalence until relatively recently. During the 1970s, the influence of the modern feminist movement led to a series of reforms designed to strengthen legislation and practice in response to physical and sexual assaults against women by intimate partners and others (National Research Council and Institute of Medicine, 1998). Since then, many legal sanction strategies have been implemented in an effort to reduce violence against women (see Gosselin, 2000; National Research Council and Institute of Medicine, 1998; Fagan, 1996; Pleck, 1989, 1987). These interventions cover nearly every aspect of the legal system—from the creation of special law enforcement, prosecution, and victim service units for intimate-partner violence and rape; to the adoption of pro-arrest policies; to the adoption of new kinds of protection orders for women being abused or stalked and the development of special courts for handling cases of intimate-partner violence.

Most legal strategies have not been rigorously evaluated, however. The evaluation literature on legal interventions is characterized by small study samples, legal problems in implementing some reforms, and difficult-to-overcome ethical problems in implementing experimental designs, among other problems (National Research Council and Institute of Medicine, 1998). The National Research Council's Committee on the Assessment of Family Violence Interventions found that no standard existed for conducting research on the immediate effects of legal reforms or on levels of subsequent abuse by offenders. The committee concluded that "accordingly, policies and procedures reflect ideology and stakeholder interests more than empirical knowledge" (National Research Council and Institute of Medicine, 1998:159). For example, few of these strategies, or their evaluations, have been guided by an explicit formulation of deterrence theory.

In a review of research assessing the impact of statutory reforms on responses by the criminal justice system, Maxwell and Post (2002) found that in general, statutory reforms increased official compliance across a number of domains, including reporting behavior, arrests, and conviction rates, and victims received improved treatment by criminal justice officials. As noted above, however, very little research has been conducted on the relationship between legislative changes and measurable reductions in the incidence of violence against women. While analyses of data from both the National Crime Victimization Survey and the Uniform Crime Reports show a decline for all violent victimization and an increase in the reporting of rape, it is not clear how the drop in rape or the increase in the reporting of rape is related to specific efforts to prevent rape or to other factors leading to general decreases in crime.

Legal Reforms for Sexual Assault

Maxwell and Post (2002) identify three areas in which legislative changes to address sexual assault have occurred since enactment of the 1970s rape statutes: sex offender notification laws, sexually violent predator laws, and laws on the use of intoxicants that facilitate sexual assault. Since 1975, all 50 states have changed their rape laws (Loh, 1981). Since the 1980s, the most broadly implemented changes have been the sex offender community notification laws, which require certain convicted sex offenders to register with law enforcement agencies and provide for community notification of the offender's presence, depending on a predefined degree of risk that these persons will reoffend. Yet little research exists on the general or specific deterrent effects of these laws. Results of a study assessing the State of Washington's notification law suggest that community notification had "little effect on recidivism as measured by new arrests for sex offenses or other types of criminal behavior" (Schram and Milloy, 1995:3). Maxwell and Post caution, however, that longer follow-up periods are needed, as well as a more qualitative assessment of changes in law enforcement and community behavior as a result of these laws.

By 1998, 12 states had enacted statutes authorizing the confinement and treatment of highly dangerous sex offenders following completion of their criminal sentence (Lieb and Matson, 1998); by 2000, an estimated 900 sex offenders were confined in the United States based on a court determination of the future danger they posed (Goldberg, 2001). Maxwell and Post (2002) were unable to find any published studies demonstrating the incapacitative effects of these predator confinement laws.

A final set of legal reforms has addressed incidents involving the use of intoxicants that facilitate sexual assault, known collectively as "date rape" drugs. By 2001, 20 states had passed legislation criminalizing the use of such drugs (State Legislature, 2001), and the U.S Congress had passed two acts prohibiting their use.

Legal Reforms for Intimate-Partner Violence

Most state legislatures have presumptive arrest laws, and many police departments prescribe that officers arrest a suspect whenever they have probable cause that a misdemeanor or felony assault has occurred between two intimate partners, even if they have not witnessed the event (Zorza, 1992; Hirschel et al., 1991; Sherman and Cohen, 1989). By 1997, more than $1 billion was being spent annually by the federal government to encourage local authorities to use formal interventions, such as arrests and prosecutions, rather than informal interventions to address intimate-partner violence (National Institute of Justice, 1997). Between 2000 and 2002, the government spent an additional $492 million to help local governments strengthen their law enforcement, prosecution, and victim services to address violence against women. Maxwell and Post (2002) were unable to find any published research evaluating changes in the incidence of intimate-partner violence as a result of the general deterrent effects of such legislation, however.

It is clear that to mount programs that work to prevent both initial and subsequent acts of violence against women, the nation must do a better job of supporting high-quality, scientific evaluation of prevention strategies and programs. Current funding levels are inadequate to support the experimental and prospective designs that would move the field forward in these areas. The committee recommends that Congress provide adequate funds to support rigorous research designs and long-term evaluations of prevention and treatment programs. Because of inherent conflicts of interest (no program wants to be found ineffective), funds for program evaluation should be independent of program funds so that the ability to evaluate interventions will not be constrained by legislative or other administrative requirements or by political interests affecting program funds or agencies. The committee also believes it is important to link health, education, and criminal justice prevention efforts, and recommends that the National Institutes of Health and the National Institute of Justice (NIJ) collaborate to develop an integrated program of rigorous evaluations of prevention, intervention, and control strategies in the area of violence against women.

Summary

There are now many educational programs designed to address the distal causes of violence against women, but there is little evidence on long-term positive attitude changes induced by these programs or on the programs' ability to reduce the incidence of violence against women. This lack of evidence of efficacy exists because evaluations cannot use victimization rates or offending patterns as measures given the poor data available on prevalence (see Chapter 2). The few evaluations that have included behavior measures have shown no difference between treatment groups. Thus at this time, it is fair to conclude that we do not know whether these programs have directly reduced violence against women. At the same time, however, evaluations of similar efforts focused on crime in general have revealed that strategies aimed at reducing opportunity are promising preventive tools. Moreover, a significant amount of research has shown that self-defense measures have been effective in preventing violence against women. In the long run, however, a permanent reduction in violence against women must rely on changing the motivations for such behaviors.

Finally, in accordance with principles of evidence-based practice, the committee recommends that evaluation of initiatives and programs to reduce violence against women be required. These evaluations should meet the scientific standards required for impact studies, including those of experimental designs. Such studies should explore whether issues exist that are particular or distinctive to evaluations of programs for violence against women. While rigorous evaluation may pose risks to a program's continued operation, assessment of outcomes is necessary to show which approaches work and whether ineffective strategies can be turned into programs that work. Moreover, such evaluations can ensure that well-intentioned programs are not actually doing harm. Government agencies such as CDC and NIJ should continue to promote research in areas in which there is insufficient evidence for making decisions about specific interventions.

RESEARCH ON DETERRENCE

The general literature on crime control provides substantial evidence that criminal justice sanctions have a deterrent effect on a wide range of behaviors. Both Nagin (1998) and Cook (1980) have found that the collective actions of the criminal justice system have a large and important deterrent effect on crime. This finding also appears to hold true—at least for the effects of arrest—for violence against women (Maxwell et al., 2001). However, Nagin (1998) notes that there is almost no empirical knowledge base regarding the extent to which any specific policy, added to the existing sanctions designed to address a specific problem, can be expected to have the desired preventive effect. He posits that in general, the response of crime rates to a change in sanction policy will depend on a number of important variables: (1) the specific form of the policy, (2) the context of its implementation, (3) the process by which people come to learn of it, (4) differences among people in their perceptions of the changes in risks and rewards resulting from the policy, and (5) feedback effects triggered by the policy itself (Nagin 1998:4).

Measuring Declarative and Deterrent Effects

Declarative effects of laws and their enforcement involve establishing normative social boundaries and distinguishing behaviors that are tolerated from those that are not. Bonnie (1981) found that laws against drug use may generate declarative effects because such laws express social disapproval. Similarly, the very existence of laws against intimate-partner violence and other violence against women symbolizes and reinforces social norms against such behavior. By shaping beliefs and attitudes toward these kinds of acts, these laws may have an effect on assaultive behavior toward women, separate from the deterrent effect of actually imposing sanctions.

Such effects are difficult to isolate and therefore to measure because they often cannot be distinguished from deterrent effects or disentangled from the effects of preexisting social norms (National Research Council, 2001). For example, some studies show that people worry about the shame and embarrassment of violating certain strongly held social norms that are supported by laws requiring compliance (see Institute of Medicine, 1999; Grasmick et al., 1991). The imposition of formal sanctions can sometimes increase compliance with a strongly held social norm beyond the levels dictated by declarative effects. However, some studies show that formal-sanction policies may lose their preventive power over time (Sherman, 1990; Ross, 1982). The committee believes that future research should explore how to gauge declarative effects and disentangle them from other types of effects.

General Deterrence

General deterrence is the impact of legal sanctions on the larger population—that is, those who have neither violated the law nor been punished. Presumably, sanctions against committing violence against women should depress prevalence and incidence, but because of continuity and definition problems in the prevalence literature, it is difficult to measure trends in this area. Nagin (1998) reviews a large literature (the data for which are assembled from surveys) focused on the links between perceptions of the risk and severity of sanctions and self-reported crime and delinquency. He notes that individuals who perceive high sanction risks and costs generally report lower criminality. With respect to violence against women, Williams and Conniff (2002) examine a number of related studies of general deterrence bearing on the perceived risk of arrest for wife assault, as well as the costs of that legal sanction, as perceived by respondents. Data were collected from a nationally representative sample of households. The authors conclude that:

- A higher perceived risk of arrest is associated with a lower likelihood of wife assault (Lackey and Williams, 1995; Williams and Hawkins, 1989a; Carmody and Williams, 1988).
- The perceived costs of arrest appear to be linked more strongly to the indirect and negative social and personal consequences of arrest than to the direct legal consequences of this sanction, such as time in jail (Williams and Hawkins, 1989b).
- Fear of arrest is a function more of the social and personal costs associated with this legal sanction itself than of the costs connected with perpetrating an act of wife assault (Williams and Hawkins, 1992).
- The perceived social costs of arrest not only are inversely related to participation in wife assault, but also are a function of other theoretically relevant factors, such as gender, race, socioeconomic status, normative approval of violence, power imbalances in heterosexual intimate relationships, and isolation from community resources of social control (Williams, 1992).

These findings provide some empirical support for a theory of general deterrence and its application to the understanding and prevention of violence against women. Williams and Conniff (2002:7) report, "*threats* of legal sanctions may well deter would-be male perpetrators of intimate-partner violence; yet this conclusion must be tempered by other implications of these findings." They believe that the nexus between legal sanctions (e.g., arrest) and informal sources of control (e.g., social costs of arrest) must be thoroughly understood. "Integrated into a larger network of social control, sanction threats may reveal their power," they note (Williams and Conniff, 2002:7). For example, a man who is enmeshed in social networks of intimate relationships, strong familial and friendship ties, work and financial gain, and other accoutrements of "conventional" living has much to lose by having his violence dramatized publicly through an arrest. This life-disrupting event could send shock waves rippling through his life, with damaging results. However, a man on the margins of conventional life may have less to lose and may well perceive arrest for wife assault, or other infractions of the law for that matter, as something that just happens, meaning little stigma is attached to getting arrested.

Specific Deterrence

Most empirical studies evaluating the effectiveness of actual experiences with sanctions in preventing or reducing violence were not explicitly designed to test the theory of specific deterrence. Nonetheless, specific deterrence is implied by the research focus on actual sanctioning experiences. Virtually all of the specific deterrence research on violence against women is on repeat intimate-partner violence.

Arrest Research

Few studies have had as much impact on violence prevention and control policies as the Minneapolis Domestic Violence Experiment (see, e.g., Sherman and Cohen, 1989). Using police records and victim interviews, the investigators in this study found that arrested suspects were significantly less likely to repeat their assaults in the 6-month follow-up period than those asked to leave the residence or those offered advice. The Spouse Assault Replication Program, funded by NIJ, replicated this research in five locations. Two studies reported evidence generally consistent with the findings of the Minneapolis study (Berk et al., 1992; Pate and Hamilton, 1992); the others reported evidence of escalation rather than deterrent effects of arrest (Hirschel et al., 1991; Sherman et al., 1992; Dunford et al., 1990). Moreover, some studies found that estimated effects were contingent on the "social bonding" of suspects, with arrest decreasing repeat violence for those who were married and employed, but increasing such violence for those who were unmarried and unemployed (for summaries, see Sherman, 1992a; Schmidt and Sherman, 1993).

Interpreting these mixed results has been problematic (see, e.g., Garner et al., 1995; Garner and Maxwell, 2000). Recent research involved pooling data from all five sites to standardize the intervention, outcome measures, and statistical models (Maxwell et al., 2001). Using victim interviews as outcome measures, this reanalysis found that independent of site, length of time between initial and follow-up interviews, and suspect characteristics, offenders in the arrested group were significantly less likely to repeat their aggression than those in the nonarrest group. However, no statistically significant effects of arrest were found when prevalence and frequency measures were based on officially recorded aggression.

Other Policing Research

Other recent research on the relationship between arrest and violence against women has focused on issues of policing rather than on the specific deterrence of police action or inaction. Feder (1998) found police were more likely to make an arrest when the assault did not involve an intimate relationship, and therefore concluded that police generally underenforce domestic violence laws. Connolly and colleagues (2000) found that arrest was actually more likely to occur in intimate situations. Chaney and Saltzstein (1998) report that direct orders requiring arrest in the form of state and local laws were effective at increasing the likelihood that officers would arrest, while Kane (1999) notes that risk to the victim was the most important factor affecting an arrest decision.

Prosecution Research

Most research on the prosecution of violence against women in recent years has focused on the issue of gaining the cooperation of victims (Robbins, 1999; Blair, 1996; Hanna, 1996). Studies have examined factors influencing the decision to prosecute (e.g., Hirschel and Hutchison, 2001; Goodman et al., 1999; Cretney and Davis, 1997; Ford, 1991). However, none of this research builds on the earlier studies of prosecution that tracked behavioral outcomes (e.g., Ford and Regoli, 1992; Fagan, 1989). As was found for arrest, Fagan (1989) reports that in cases where prosecution was attempted, convictions obtained, and offenders sentenced, reductions in subsequent violence were greatest for less-severe offenders. However, for offenders with "more severe histories of violence, the imposition of more severe sanctions was associated with increased incidence of violence" (Fagan, 1989:384). Ford and Regoli (1992) report similar findings. They note that these mixed results do suggest that serious offenders are less influenced by legal sanctions, and indeed if such sanctions have any influence at all, they may actually increase violence against women (Mills, 1998).

Summary

The literature on repeat intimate-partner violence demonstrates that legal sanctions do have deterrent effects, although modest in magnitude, but that these effects vary by the characteristics of perpetrators, their relationship with their partners, their stake in social conformity, and factors influencing the decision to impose sanctions. Future research on this topic should seek to fill gaps in the research on general deterrence that may have implications for more-successful policies and practices. Factors that may moderate the effects of sanction risks and experiences on the violent victimization of women include neighborhood and community characteristics (see, e.g., Fagan, 1996), and especially the life circumstances of women victims (e.g., Bowman, 1992; Frisch, 1992; Lerman, 1992; Zorza,

1992) (see also Chapter 3). Moreover, such research should focus on all forms of violence against women, not just intimate-partner violence.

A BROADER FRAMEWORK FOR FUTURE RESEARCH

While research shows that the collective actions of the criminal justice system exert a substantial deterrent effect on crime, this fact is of limited value in formulating policy for specific crime problems (Nagin, 1998). It is the committee's view that future research on deterring violence against women would be of most benefit if folded into broader efforts to study the decision making of potential perpetrators and the deterrence of criminal behavior generally. This is a particularly important point given the scope and cost of program efforts aimed at deterring and preventing violence against women. The committee identified four research gaps that impede progress in informing the development of effective policies and programs to deter and control crime. The committee believes that research in these four areas is critical to improving the ability to deter violence against women.

Long-Term Effects of Sanctioning Policy

There is a large amount of research on short-term effects of crime control policies and programs, but almost nothing is known about long-term effects. If, for example, the principal deterrent effect of formal sanctions for violence against women (or other crimes) derives from fear of social stigma, the extent to which such penalties are actually meted out could either reinforce or erode such fear. Nagin (1998:5) posits that "policies that are effective in the short-term might erode the very basis for their effectiveness in the long-term if they increase the proportion of the population that is stigmatized." A criminal record cannot be socially isolating if it is commonplace. Thus, while arrest policies appear to work in the aggregate to reduce intimate-partner violence (Maxwell et al., 2001), some research studies indicate that they have no effect, or a criminogenic effect, on some offenders (Sherman, 1992b). The committee believes that research on the ways in which social stigma for acts of intimate-partner violence is generated and then either sustained or eroded would inform the development of more-effective policies and programs.

Formation of Perceptions of the Risk of Sanctions

There is a large body of research analyzing the links between perceptions of the risk of sanctions and behavior (e.g., Lackey and Williams, 1995; Nagin and Paternoster, 1993; Bachman et al., 1992; Williams and

Hawkins, 1989a; Carmody and Williams, 1988; Paternoster et al., 1982; Grasmick and Bryjak, 1980). One study on the deterrent effect of such perceptions with regard to intimate-partner violence was described above (Williams and Conniff, 2002). However, very little is known about how these perceptions are formed. Behavioral decision theorists have found that human beings prefer more rather than less certainty about the probable outcomes of their choices. For example, where the perceived probability of punishment is uncertain, there may be an initial deterrent effect. However, Sherman found that initial deterrent effects are eroded as offenders learn through experience that they have overestimated the chances of being caught and punished (Sherman, 1992b; Ross, 1982).

This finding supports Nagin's (1998) point that although the perception of the risk that a sanction will be imposed may affect the decision to commit a crime, one cannot therefore conclude that a specific policy deters crime. To know that, one must have a more specific understanding of how risk perception is generated and sustained. For example, we do not know whether offenders perceive a risk of penalty because of the overall effectiveness of enforcement or because there is a crime-specific mechanism in place. In addition, we do not know how quickly policy changes influence perceptions of sanction risk. Better studies are also needed of the effects of the crime rate on actual sanction levels and of how those effects in turn influence the formation of perceptions of the risk of punishment. Finally, it is important to explore Sherman's (1990) theory that initial deterrence can be made permanent by continually experimenting with novel police strategies, deployments, or enforcement priorities.

How Responses to Crime Vary Across Time and Space

Many evaluations of the deterrent effects of specific policies, such as increasing the number of police, are too broad—measuring effects across the general population. Dugan and Apel's (2002) recent analysis of differential risk for different groups of women underscores the need for another strategy. Nagin (1998) found that while there may be some credible estimates of the average deterrent effects of certain policies (e.g., effects of arrest policies on intimate-partner violence), the capacity to translate those effects into a prediction for a specific place or population is limited. For purposes of deterrence, he concludes, "It is the response of crime to policy in a specific city or state that is relevant to its population, not the average response across all cities and states" (Nagin, 1998:6). This effect has been demonstrated by the approach to deterring gun violence among youth in Boston, as described and documented by Kennedy et al. (2001) and recently evaluated by Braga et al. (2001).

Links Between Actual and Intended Policy

Finally, the link between intended and actual policy has not been well explored. In some jurisdictions, for example, police have reacted to mandatory arrest policies by arresting both partners involved in intimate-partner assault calls. With regard to policy changes in the early 1980s calling for increased penalties for gun carrying, the court in one city and the police in another found ways to circumvent the change so the system could essentially maintain the status quo. Arrest or sentencing policies may be circumvented in other ways—through plea bargaining, for example. There is a need for research on how sanctions are generated and implemented so their effects on crime and on perceptions of the risk of sanctions can be better understood.

5

Identifying and Treating Offenders

O ver the past four decades, efforts to determine what motivates men to commit crimes of violence against women have not led to definitive answers. While past research focused on sexual assault, recent research examines battery and homicide against intimate partners. New evidence from longitudinal studies connects developmental problems, such as early conduct disorder, to later violence against women (Moffitt et al., 2001). In addition, researchers are formulating theories to categorize rapists, batterers, and other types of individuals who victimize women and others and exploring what treatments may help prevent offenders from repeating their behaviors.

CHARACTERISTICS OF OFFENDERS

Motivations of Men Who Rape

Explanations for why men rape range from individual determinants—such as physiology and neurophysiology, personality traits, attitudes, alcohol abuse, and psychopathology—to sex and power motives, social learning theories, dyadic contexts, institutional influences, societal influences, and multifactorial models (for a review see National Research Council, 1996). The two most common explanations are that rape is sexually motivated or motivated by a desire for power. However, it has generally been accepted that multiple causal factors are involved in sexually aggressive behavior (National Research Council, 1996).

Most researchers and clinical investigators agree that sexual offenders are a heterogeneous group with differing motivations. The development of taxonomies based on these differences may enhance the efficacy of clinical decisions and provide guidance for the study of etiology, recidivism, and the life-span adaptation of sexual offenders. Knight and Prentky (1990) developed one such taxonomy of rapists by identifying specific categories of offenders common to available typologies and determining type-defining variables. Their model identifies nine types of rapists falling into one of four descriptive summary categories based on motivation: opportunistic, pervasively angry, sexual, and vindictive.

For opportunistic rapists, sexual assault was found to be an impulsive, usually unplanned, predatory act, occasioned more by contextual and immediately antecedent factors than by protracted or stylized sexual fantasy. These offenders are likely to have a life history of poor impulse control. Pervasively angry rapists are described as motivated primarily by nonsexualized, undifferentiated anger. They show gratuitous aggression, directed equally toward men and women. Sexually motivated rapists are characterized as driven by either protracted sexual or sadistic fantasies or preoccupations. Sadistic types may be overt or muted, depending on the level of aggression or physically damaging behavior they exhibit during the rape. For nonsadistic types, rape was found to be a result of sexual arousal, distorted views of women and sex, and feelings of inadequacy regarding the perpetrator's sexuality and masculine self-image. Finally, Knight and Prentky's (1990) taxonomy describes vindictive rapists as intending for the sexual assault to result in physical harm, degradation, and humiliation of the victim. Their anger and aggression are centered primarily on women.

Motivations of Men Who Batter

In most studies, wife batterers are treated as a homogeneous group. Recent research, however, indicates that men who exhibit violence toward their spouses are heterogeneous along theoretically important dimensions. Thus, developing and comparing subtypes of violent men and understanding how each subtype differs from nonviolent men may help in identifying the various underlying processes that contribute to violent behavior.

Holtzworth-Munroe and Meehan (2002) describe a typology that integrates several theories of aggression into a developmental model of differing types of violence by husbands (see also Holtzworth-Munroe and Stuart, 1994). That model highlights the importance of correlates of male violence, including both historical correlates—violence in the family of origin and association with delinquent peers, gleaned from the broader literature on delinquency—and proximal correlates—individual characteristics of violent behaviors. According to this model, batterers can be classified into three categories according to severity/frequency of marital violence, generality of violence (marital only or extrafamilial), and the batterer's psychopathology or personality disorders:

- **Family-only** batterers are predicted to engage in the least marital violence, the lowest levels of psychological and sexual abuse, and the least violence outside the home. Holtzworth-Munroe and Stuart (1994) identify little or no psychopathology in this group.
- **Dysphoric/borderline** batterers are predicted to engage in moderate to severe wife abuse, but little abuse outside of the family.
- **Violent/antisocial batterers** are predicted to engage in high levels of marital violence and the highest levels of extrafamilial violence—criminal behavior, arrests, and substance abuse.

Holtzworth-Munroe and Stuart (1994) theorize that family-only batterers engage in aggressive acts as a result of a combination of stress (personal and/or marital) and low-level risk factors, including childhood exposure to marital violence and a lack of relationship skills. After such incidents, however, the men's low levels of psychopathology and related problems (low impulsivity, low attachment dysfunction), combined with their lack of hostility toward women and lack of positive attitudes toward violence, lead to remorse and prevent an escalation of the aggression.

In contrast, Holtzworth-Munroe and Stuart hypothesize that dysphoric/borderline batterers come from backgrounds of parental abuse and rejection and therefore have difficulty forming a stable, trusting attachment with an intimate partner. Thus, these individuals tend to be highly jealous and dependent on, yet fearful, of losing their wives. Moreover, they are likely to be impulsive, lack marital skills, and have attitudes that are hostile toward women and supportive of violence. This group resembles batterers studied by Dutton (1995), who suggests that these men's early traumatic experiences lead to borderline personality organization, anger, and insecure attachment, which, when the men become frustrated, result in violence against their adult attachment figure—the wife.

Finally, generally violent/antisocial batterers are predicted to resemble other antisocial, aggressive groups. They are expected to have experienced high levels of violence in their family of origin and association with deviant peers. They are impulsive, lack skills (marital and nonmarital), have hostile attitudes toward women, and view violence as acceptable. For this category of batterers, marital violence is conceptualized as part of their general use of aggression and engagement in antisocial behavior.

Later research by Holtzworth-Munroe et al. (2000) supports this typology and adds a fourth subgroup—low-level antisocial—which falls between the family-only and generally violent/antisocial groups. This group exhibits moderate levels of antisocial behavior, general violence, and marital violence, similar to the levels predicted for the family-only group.

Recent data suggest that such typologies make it easier to understand and predict the outcomes of treatment. Jones and Gondolf (in press) report that although reassault following treatment is not predicted by batterer personality profiles, it is predicted by a history of arrest at intake and drunkenness during the follow-up period. Gondolf and White (2001) identify a wide variety of personality profiles among repeat reassaulters and note subclinical or low levels of personality dysfunction among the majority of these individuals.

A clinical implication of batterer typologies such as that described by Holtzworth-Munroe and Meehan (2002) is that treatment outcomes might be improved by matching interventions to types of batterers. For example, in a comparison of two treatment models, Saunders (1996) found that offenders with dependent personalities had significantly lower rates of recidivism than those found in other types of offenders in process-psychodynamic treatment groups, and that offenders with antisocial personalities had lower rates of recidivism in structured, feminist–cognitive–behavioral groups. Furthermore, it may be important to consider the applicability of interventions developed in other fields, such as criminal justice. For example, the potential usefulness of intensive rehabilitation supervision—close monitoring of offenders in the community, along with rehabilitation focused on criminogenic needs—is receiving attention in work with antisocial groups (Gendreau et al., 1994).

Holtzworth-Munroe and Meehan (2002) recommend that prospective, longitudinal studies be conducted to identify the developmental pathways that result in different types of violent husbands. Such studies would allow researchers to examine the constructs assumed to predict the use of violence among samples of adolescents or children, and to then observe the relationship between those variables and the emergence of relationship violence as study participants enter intimate relationships. For example, the Dunedin Multidisciplinary Health and Development Study identified developmental pathways to violent behavior, including partner violence (see Moffitt et al., 2001). Data from this study suggest that antisocial behavior is predictable across time. A developmental history of conduct problems was found to be the strongest predictor of perpetration of intimate-partner violence for both males and females (Moffitt and Caspi, 1998). This was true even when such a history was compared with previously established risk factors, such as low family socioeconomic status, conflicted early family relations, and weak childhood cognitive functioning and educational difficulties. Such longitudinal cohort studies can eliminate possible biases of retrospective studies, such as faulty memory.

The committee believes that future research should focus on learning more about perpetrators of violence generally and use this information as the context for specific studies of domestic violence. In the past, research on domestic violence has not taken theories of general violence into account, focusing instead on theories of patriarchy and power relations without considering possible explanatory variables from other disciplines or from the longitudinal literature on the development of violent behavior (National Research Council and Institute of Medicine, 1998). Research should take into account the possibility that battering is caused by a more complex set of hierarchical influences, such as weak social controls, situational arousal, and psychopathology, that cause violence in general (Fagan, 1996). The batterer typology described by Holtzworth-Munroe and Meehan (2002) shows how research on violence in general can inform research on male batterers by using a more inclusive set of variables. In addition, social ecological studies (as discussed in Chapter 3) might inform future research on batterers by linking batterer typologies with research on the social conditions that may shape various battering behaviors.

Links Between Women's Victimization and Offending

Research has shown that women who engage in violence are often victims of violence themselves. According to an analysis by the Bureau of Justice Statistics (Harlow, 1999), 45 percent of women in state prisons who had committed a violent offense reported that they had been physically or sexually abused at some time during their lives. And 37 percent of female offenders (probationers and federal and state prison and jail inmates) reported they had been physically or sexually abused before age 18—a significantly higher percentage than is reported for the general population.

In some cases, violence may be the only immediate response to danger for a threatened woman. However, Moffitt et al. (2001) report a large number of supporting analyses suggesting that women's violence against partners cannot be completely explained as defensive. In the Dunedin sample, for example, women who had engaged in partner violence were 4.4 times more likely than male offenders to have committed a violent crime against someone other than their partner.

Both theoretical and empirical models need to be expanded to enable a better understanding of such female-perpetrated violence, including any commonalities this violence may have with that perpetrated by men, as well as the violent victimization experienced over the life course by women who engage in violent behavior. Research designs should include an examination of the environments, as well as the cultural context, of violent women. More research is also needed on the increased rates of incarceration of women, changes in the percentages of women in prisons and jails for drug-related and other nonviolent offenses and for violent offenses, and the implications of these changes (Kruttschnitt and Gartner, 2003).

INTERVENTIONS

The fields of domestic violence and sexual assault have developed separately, with distinct service and research traditions. One reason for this separation is the tendency of programs for sexual offenders to target a greater variety of offender types (rapists and child molesters within and outside the family, juvenile and adult offenders). Despite this separation, the two fields share some similar treatment orientations, innovations, and controversies. As noted throughout this report, researchers and practitioners might benefit from placing their work in the broader context of violent criminals in general and discussing domestic violence and sexual assault as subtypes of general criminal offending.

Types of Treatment Programs

Programs for both domestic violence offenders and sex offenders tend to integrate several approaches through a number of phases that first expand offenders' definitions of abuse and hold them responsible for it, and then teach them alternative reactions and behaviors (Gondolf, 1997; Freeman-Longo et al., 1995). The most common format for delivering services is men's groups (Marshall, 1999), followed by individual counseling (Pirog-Good and Stets-Kealey, 1985).

Saunders and Hamill (2002) report that cognitive–behavioral approaches are especially prevalent in sex offender treatment programs, which emphasize highly specific techniques such as relapse prevention (Burton and Smith-Darden, 2001; Marshall and Serran, 2000). Such programs are also more likely than domestic violence treatment programs to explore and attempt to resolve past traumas, with more than 70 percent of the former programs focusing on childhood victimization (Burton and Smith-Darden, 2001; Freeman-Longo et al., 1995). Most interventions can be classified along several dimensions based on their underlying assumptions. Table 5-1 summarizes key features of treatment programs for domestic violence and sexual assault offenders.

TABLE 5-1 Types of Offender Treatment Programs

Program Type	Description	Underlying Assumption
Domestic Violence		
Skills training	Group members rehearse positive behaviors to build skills.	Offenders have socially learned behavioral deficits and behavioral excesses.
Cognitive approaches	Attempts to restructure faulty patterns of thinking and build awareness of core belief systems developed in childhood.	Faulty patterns of thinking lead to negative emotions, which in turn lead to abusive behavior.
Sex role resocialization	Helps men see the negative effects of constricted male roles and the benefits of gender equality (Saunders, 1984).	Rigid socialization of constricted male roles results in male dominance.
Building awareness of control tactics	Helps men take ownership of their intentions to control others (Pence and Paymar, 1994).	Abusive men use isolation, demeaning language, control of finances, and other means to control their victims.
Family systems approaches	Analyze and change communication patterns of couples.	Couples unknowingly engage in repeated cycles of interaction that may culminate in abuse (Neidig et al., 1984).
Trauma-based approaches	Attempt to resolve childhood traumas, in particular the traumas of witnessing parental violence and being physically abused by parents (Browne, Saunders, and Staecker, 1997).	Abusive men cannot empathize well with others because they are cut off from their own painful memories of childhood traumas.
Sexual Assault		
Comprehensive evaluation and risk assessment	Analyze abusive behavior to identify warning signs and prevent future offending.	Offenders engage in a chain of thoughts, feelings, stimuli, and behavior that leads to an offense.
Psycho-social-sexual education	Program staff use a structured curriculum to work with the offender and family members to prepare him for treatment and enhance the ultimate impact of other intervention components.	

Continued

TABLE 5-1 Continued

Program Type	Description	Underlying Assumption
Process treatment	Sex offense–specific individual, group, and family therapies are used to achieve honesty, responsibility, empathy, and remorse.	
Focused treatment	Trains the abuser to gain control over specific acts of offending and to rehearse the skills necessary to maintain recovery.	Offenders have low impulse control in specific situations.
Behavioral supervision	Monitors and controls the abuser's everyday living environment to minimize his opportunity to reoffend and teach him internal control.	Opportunity increases the likelihood of offending.
Case management	Manages interventions with the abuser along the continuum of care so that accountability and participation in offense-specific treatment are ensured, and the offender's placement in the least-restrictive safe setting is maintained.	
Medication	Some form of medication, usually antiandrogens, is used in about half the programs in conjunction with other methods (Burton and Smith-Darden, 2001).	Medication can reduce sexual urges in the most compulsive offenders.

SOURCE: Saunders and Hamill (2002).

Outcome Studies

Research on treatment outcomes has only begun to emerge and is in general of poor quality. Past evaluations have been nonexperimental and therefore unable to rule out nontreatment effects, or have used reports of official records, which are likely to greatly underestimate rates of violence. Many studies also have not included sufficient follow-up periods to measure recidivism or other long-term outcomes, nor have such outcomes been uniformly identified, conceptualized, and operationalized (problems with evaluation studies are discussed by Gondolf, 2001, 1997; Marques, 1999; McConaghy, 1999; Holtzworth-Munroe et al., 1995; Tolman and Edleson, 1995; Hamberger and Hastings, 1993; and Rosenfeld, 1992).

Domestic Violence

Saunders and Hamill (2002) report that few of the more than 30 studies of program effectiveness they reviewed had rigorous designs that would allow for firm conclusions (see reviews by Babcock et al., in press; Davis and Taylor, 1999; and Tolman and Edleson, 1995). More-rigorous evaluations tend to use experimental designs and longer follow-up periods (e.g., 1 to 4 years). These studies have suggested that the structure of treatment groups and the length of treatment may influence the effectiveness of treatment (Edleson and Syers, 1991, 1990), that treatment over a longer time span may be more effective than that over a shorter period (Davis et al., 2000), and that the success of certain treatments may depend on the typology of the offenders (Saunders, 1996). Experimental studies have revealed no differences in outcome between couples' groups and men's groups, although both have been associated with significant reductions in abuse (O'Leary et al., 1999; Brannen and Rubin, 1996). Nor have differences in outcome been found among four types of treatment involving male naval personnel: cognitive–behavioral men's groups, cognitive–behavioral "quasi-couples groups" (low partner attendance), rigorous monitoring, and stabilization and safety planning (pretreatment screening, safety planning, and referrals for women) (Dunford, 2000). Meta-analyses using partner and official reports indicated that the effects of treatment were small (Babcock et al., in press; Levesque, 1998).

Sexual Abuse

Saunders and Hamill (2002) report the results of several recent meta-analyses of outcomes of sex offender treatment programs. The most rigorous such analysis, coordinated by the Association for the Treatment of Sexual Abusers, involved 42 studies of psychological treatment in both community and institutional settings (Hanson et al., 2000). Of those who received treatment, 12 percent had committed another sexual offense, versus 18 percent in comparison groups; for any type of offense, the rates were 29 and 42 percent, respectively. For the 15 most rigorous studies, the sexual offense recidivism rates were 10 percent for the treated and 17 percent for the untreated offenders. Both institutional and community-based treatments were associated with lower rates of recidivism.

Many programs supplement individual and group therapy with medications that lower the level of testosterone. These medications provide relief to some compulsive sex offenders (Robinson and Valcour, 1995; Fedoroff et al., 1992), but their mandated use is controversial (Miller, 1998; Prentky, 1997). Prentky (1997) cautions strongly against this approach as an exclusive treatment for sexual aggressors.

Areas for further research that may prove fruitful include matching of offender types to types of treatment and matching of treatment to the motivational stage of the offender. Recognition of how types of offenders differ along key theoretical dimensions, such as developmental background, social context, and mental disorder, should be part of the conceptual development and testing of offender interventions (Fagan, 1996).

Improving Quality-of-Outcome Studies

Most offender treatment programs have been based on theoretical assumptions, but their outcomes are as yet unclear. The committee recommends that improvements be made to the quality of outcome studies and that all treatment programs be evaluated. Saunders and Hamill (2002) provide suggestions for such improvements. First, evaluations should include a comprehensive set of outcome measures and develop ways of reducing the possibility of faked improvements. Second, they should provide evidence on whether the treatments proposed were actually the ones delivered; this could be done by standardizing treatments through use of a manual, by providing close supervision, or by employing other approaches that can demonstrate treatment integrity. Third, evaluations should also include information on participant selection into treatment and attrition during and after treatment, as both methodological concerns affect the generalizability of study findings. Offenders who enter and complete treatment, especially voluntary programs and court-mandated programs that do not have consequences for noncompliance, may differ in important ways from offenders who do not. Finally, program evaluations should use experimental designs involving comparison or control groups whenever possible if firm conclusions are to be drawn.

Reducing Program Attrition

One of the biggest problems in working with offenders is the high rate of attrition in treatment programs. Saunders and Hamill (2002) note that men who engage in domestic violence and sexual assault have little desire to participate in treatment programs, even when the programs are court-ordered or could lead to an earlier end to incarceration, and only a small percentage enroll in treatment voluntarily.

Several methods have been proposed for reducing program attrition. One approach involves a coordinated community-wide response that includes criminal justice sanctions; although most available evidence does not demonstrate that this approach keeps men in treatment, evidence suggests that criminal justice mandates may help reduce attrition among younger, less-educated men (Daly and Pelowski, 2000; Saunders and Parker, 1989). One method that has had some success in improving retention is the use of a marathon orientation group—a 12-hour group session designed to provide an overview of upcoming treatment, as well as to teach concrete skills (Tolman and Bhosley, 1991). Another promising innovation uses video and discussion to facilitate the development of feelings of compassion (Stosny, 1994). More-traditional approaches that rely on supportive phone calls and handwritten notes from therapists at the outset of treatment and after any missed sessions have also been shown to be related to continuation in treatment (Taft et al., 2001).

Most convicted sex offenders who reside in the community are mandated to participate in treatment programs as a condition of probation or parole. Increasingly, probation and parole departments are using specially trained personnel to supervise sex offenders (English et al., 1996). Whether these methods actually decrease attrition is not known.

Assessing Dangerousness and Risk of Recidivism

A variety of instruments have been developed to assess the likelihood that an offender will engage in additional battering or sexual assault after completion of a treatment program, although the predictive validity of these instruments has not been established (Dutton and Kropp, 2000; Roehl and Guertin, 2000; Websdale, 2000). Practitioners in programs for domestic violence offenders may be required to warn or protect potential victims if they believe lethal violence is imminent (Hart, 1988; McNeill, 1987). They may also be asked to make predictions about the recurrence of severe violence in order to provide specialized treatment or recommend closer supervision.

Campbell's (1986) Danger Assessment instrument for use with battered women is a 15-item checklist that correlates with violence severity and distinguishes between victims who go to emergency rooms and those who do not (Campbell, 1995). MOSAIC-20 (de Becker, 1997) emphasizes the role of the survivor's intuition, which some evidence suggests is an accurate way to predict severe violence (Weisz et al., 2000). More research is needed to determine the predictive usefulness of survivor's intuition.

Other risk assessment tools focus on the risk of recidivism. The Spousal Assault Risk Assessment Guide (Kropp et al., 1999) uses reports from as many sources as possible, including interviews with offenders and victims, official records, and standardized tests. The Domestic Violence Inventory relies on a questionnaire administered to offenders and contains the following subscales: truthfulness, alcohol use, control, drug use, violence, and coping with stress (Risk and Needs Assessment, 1996).

Research on the prediction of recidivism by sex offenders has led to the creation of at least 24 measures of the offender's personal and legal history, including offender's age, victim's age and gender, and details of the offenses (Doren, 1999). Of the 24 risk assessment measures identified by Doren, however, only 8 have been validated for assessing the risk of reoffending. The use of statistically validated measures as opposed to clinical intuition is viewed as increasingly important because the former are usually more accurate. Of the measures frequently used in the evaluation of sex offenders, a recent study of predictive validity showed that the Violence Risk Appraisal Guide, RRASOR, and Static-99 were best at predicting sexual recidivism (Barbaree et al., 2001). Research on predicting sex offender recidivism may benefit from the more-general research on risk prediction devices for serious offending (see, e.g., Lattimore et al., 1995).

Culturally Competent Interventions

Many newly developed programs are addressing the diverse cultural backgrounds of clients (Lewis, 1999; Marshall et al., 1998). It is posited that treatment programs might be more successful if the cultural and world views of clients were better supported by treatment models and clinicians' knowledge base (Jones et al., 1999). Subcultural mistrust of the dominant culture, help-seeking patterns in collectivist cultures, and subcultural communication styles might better explain resistance to treatment than intrapsychic mechanisms (Lewis, 1999). However, the committee could find no assessments of the effectiveness of such programs compared with treatment programs that do not specifically consider cultural factors.

Williams and Becker (1994) distinguish among "color-blind" programs that do not take race or ethnicity into account, "culturally focused" programs that pay attention to historical and contemporary experiences of particular cultural groups, and "culturally centered" programs that place a particular culture at the center of treatment and use culturally significant rituals. Some programs give men the choice of same-race or mixed-race groups. In addition to the Afrocentric models being developed by Williams (1994), programs are available for Southeast Asians, Native Americans, Latinos, and other ethnic and racial groups (Carrillo and Tello, 1998; Healey et al., 1998). Saunders and Hamill (2002) note that evaluations of efforts to coordinate and consult with the minority community should provide useful guidance, and they recommend that qualitative research on same-race groups be extended to further assess the impact of these groups on treatment attrition and outcome.

CONCLUSIONS

More research is needed on treatment for perpetrators of violence against women. Possible subjects for future research include matching of what is known about different types of offenders to appropriate interventions, methods to reduce program attrition, the usefulness of risk assessment tools and survivor's intuition in predicting recidivism, and increased attention to training in cultural competence and the use of culturally specific interventions. Research should also address women who commit violent acts, and should further explore interactions between women's experiences of violent victimization and their own violent offending.

Despite an accumulation of studies evaluating programs for domestic violence offenders, rigorous studies are few, and firm conclusions about the effectiveness of interventions cannot be drawn. The quality of outcome studies needs to be improved for all treatment programs.

6

The Future of Research on Violence Against Women: Final Thoughts

The Department of Justice and the Department of Health and Human Services have supported research on violence against women for over two decades. Findings have had a significant impact—perhaps more than in any other crime-related topic—on legislation, criminal justice policy, and, to a lesser extent, health policy at all levels of government. Much of what has been accomplished has been driven by a cadre of dedicated researchers and nongovernmental groups advocating for the safety of women and girls.

The committee found that while much has been accomplished, a great deal of work remains to be done. Federal agencies have made a very promising start in carrying out the research agenda delineated in *Understanding Violence Against Women* (National Research Council, 1996), and the committee recommends that those efforts continue. However, because of the comparatively low level of funding that has been available for rigorous studies on violence against women (compared, for example, with drug abuse and other health or behavioral areas), federal research agencies have tended to fund important but less expensive studies instead of developing the research infrastructure required to support studies on causes of violence against women and the impact of interventions. The prevention and treatment studies discussed in this volume would all have benefited from better data from surveys and longitudinal studies. The committee wishes to emphasize the importance of building a research infrastructure that can support sophisticated studies on the causes, nature, and scope of violence against women and the kinds of interventions that will prevent or reduce such violence in the future. Therefore, top priority for the immediate future should be given to improving definitions and the quality of data in surveys, conducting longitudinal studies of violence against women, and evaluating theoretically sound prevention and intervention programs.

IMPROVING DEFINITIONS AND DATA

Understanding Violence Against Women calls for improvements in research methods, including the development of clear definitions by researchers and practitioners of the terms used in their work, and the development and testing of (new) scales and other measurement tools to make operational the key and most-used definitions. While some new work has been funded in this most critical of areas, the committee believes that a more coordinated and continuous research strategy would help remedy the measurement problems discussed in this report. Without consistency in the use of terms across studies, research in this field will remain fragmented; new measurement instruments that have been developed may not receive adequate testing or experimental use in studies that can demonstrate their power; and accurate prevalence and incidence estimates, especially of severe violence, will remain elusive.

One avenue the committee has recommended for accomplishing such improvements is to investigate how to link existing datasets, such as those found in Table 2-1, and how to link information from these datasets with findings from clinical and longitudinal research. Such an effort would provide more immediate information on the risks of, responses to, and consequences of violence against women and perhaps on the impact of interventions as well. The formulation of a new framework for developing standard definitions to overcome the lack of conceptual and operational clarity that currently exists would be a critical part of this effort, and could address other problems as well, such as differences in sample selection among surveys and studies. The steering committee believes that the federal research agencies responsible for developing research and statistics in this area are best positioned to develop a process for designing this framework. For example, the Bureau of Justice Statistics had relatively recent experience salient to such an effort in the research process that informed the redesign of the National Crime Victimization Survey.

The recommended effort to improve definitions would also inform any new undertaking to provide better national survey data on violence against women. The problems with survey data on violence against women have been well documented in this report. The committee believes that the program of research described above for assessing what can be learned from extant data sources would provide important information on prevalence and on how best to proceed in developing more-accurate datasets and prevalence estimates—especially whether a new and continuous national survey is needed. If it is determined that such a survey is needed, Congress should provide the additional funding necessary to support data collection and analysis, and to make the data available to the academic community for research and to the public. If we are to advance the state of knowledge on violence against women, there can be no higher priority than improving data on prevalence and incidence. Without improved data, we cannot determine whether the programs that are being implemented under the Violence Against Women Act of 1994 or under other auspices or funding streams are having the desired effect of reducing violence against women.

CONDUCTING LONGITUDINAL STUDIES

The committee found credible evidence from an existing New Zealand longitudinal study (Moffitt et al., 2001) that perpetrators of violence against women commonly have histories of violence and conduct problems outside of intimate relationships, and that the same is true for women who commit violent acts. The committee agrees with workshop presenters and attendees that information from longitudinal studies of U.S. populations is needed to examine the causes and consequences of violence against and by women, especially to determine which risk factors are truly unique to lethal outcomes or those involving severe injury. Studies that address risk factors for women should have female respondents, but longitudinal population-based studies that include both men and women also are critical. The National Institute of Justice (NIJ) already has funded some secondary analyses of existing longitudinal studies that may yet prove fruitful for this purpose. Longitudinal studies currently in progress, such as the Project on Human Development in Chicago Neighborhoods, might be able to provide some of this information, an option worth exploring before generating an expensive new longitudinal study. The committee recognizes that additional funding would be needed for longitudinal studies on violence against women, and recommends that the National Institutes of Health and NIJ should collaborate on the design and implementation of such studies so that both criminal justice and health issues will be adequately addressed.

EVALUATING PREVENTION AND INTERVENTION PROGRAMS

Many programs have been implemented to prevent and deter violence against women over the last two decades. As this report demonstrates, however, few credible evaluations of the efficacy of these programs have been conducted. This lack of program evaluation is attributable in part to inadequate past and current levels of funding, which cannot support the kinds of experimental approaches needed to determine impact; in part to the lack of good data to support strong nonexperimental research designs; and in part to the lack of independence of many research and evaluation studies from the programs or approaches being evaluated. There may be other factors mitigating against strong evaluation studies as well. If we are to be able to determine whether programs are working, having no effect, or doing harm, more rigorous evaluation studies and the funding and infrastructure required to support them should be a priority of federal research agencies conducting studies on violence against women.

OTHER EMERGING RESEARCH PRIORITIES

Understanding Violence Against Women recommends that all research on violence against women take into account the context within which women live their lives and in which the violence occurs and that this context include social, cultural, and individual factors. Work on neighborhood context has only begun to emerge, however. Similarly, research on legal reforms and sanctions indicates that both have a deterrent effect on reoffending for intimate-partner violence, and some of these reforms may have a general deterrent effect as well. Some work has been funded in these areas, and the committee recommends that these studies continue.

Social Ecology Studies

As noted in Chapter 3, the spatial concentration of crime is apparent on any urban map using any measure, including gun crime, gang crime, drug selling, or violence against women. These facts confirm earlier findings by Shaw and McKay (1942) that crime persists in certain places over generations and despite demographic changes, and have led to a new focus in general crime studies on place-centered analysis.

Social ecological factors may affect not only rates of violence, but also the efficacy of legal sanctions and social interventions. A new program of research on these issues is needed to address important aspects of neighborhood and community life and their implications for violence against women. For example, research should address how individual factors and area conditions interact to affect rates of violence against women, the interdependence of violence against women and violence against men in the same social areas, whether the availability of and access to local services can affect localized violence rates, and whether sanctions may be differentially effective by locale (see, e.g., Sampson and Bartusch, 1998).

Deterrence Studies

The committee found that legal reforms and sanctions have both a specific deterrent effect on those who have already offended and a general deterrent effect for intimate-partner violence. Future deterrence research should build upon existing studies on intimate-partner violence, with an expanded focus that includes other types of violence against women. Research is needed on the long-term effects of sanctioning policy, on how offenders form perceptions of the risk of punishment, on the extent to which levels of violence against women respond to policy in specific locations, and on the links between intended policy and the policy that is actually implemented and its effect on levels of violence.

Finally, there is emerging and credible evidence that the general origins and behavioral patterns of various forms of violence, such as male violence against women and men and female violence against men and women, may be similar. The committee believes that while gender-based studies of violence against women are important, some level of integration of research is critical to advancing our understanding of the causes of violence against and by women. Integrating studies of violence against women with the larger literature on crime and violence would enrich both bodies of research intellectually, and provide a more comprehensive basis for violence prevention and deterrence strategies.

References

CHAPTER 1

Capaldi, D.M., and S. Clark
 1998   Prospective family predictors of aggression toward female partners for young at-
        risk young men. *Developmental Psychology* 34:1175-1188.
Craven, D.
 1997   *Sex Differences in Violent Victimization, 1994.* Washington, DC: Bureau of Justice
        Statistics. Available online at http://www.ojp.usdoj.gov/bjs/pub/pdf/sdvv.pdf
        [accessed April 4, 2003].
Farrington, D.
 1994   Childhood, adolescent, and adult features of violent males. In *Aggressive Behavior:
        Current Perspectives*, L.R. Huesmann, ed. New York: Plenum Press.
Felson, R.B.
 2002   *Violence and Gender Reexamined.* Washington, DC: American Psychological Asso-
        ciation.
Ford, D.A., R. Bachman, M. Friend, and M. Meloy
 2002   *Controlling Violence Against Women: A Research Perspective on the 1994 VAWA's
        Criminal Justice Impacts.* Washington, DC: National Institute of Justice, U.S. De-
        partment of Justice.
Fox, J., and M. Zawitz
 2002   *Homicide Trends in the United States.* Washington, DC: Bureau of Justice Statistics.
        Available online at http://www.ojp.usdoj.gov/bjs/homicide/homtrnd.htm [ac-
        cessed August 1, 2003].
Giordano, P.C., T.J. Millhollin, S.A. Cernkovich, and M.D. Pugh
 1999   Delinquency, identity, and women's involvement in relationship violence. *Crimi-
        nology* 37:17-40.
Holtzworth-Munroe, A., and J.C. Meehan
 2002   *Typologies of Maritally Violent Men: A Summary of Current Knowledge and Sugges-
        tions for Future Research.* Paper prepared for the Workshop on Issues in Research
        on Violence Against Women, The National Academies, Washington, DC, January
        3-4.

Moffitt, T.E., A. Caspi, M. Rutter, and P. Silva
  2001   *Sex Differences in Antisocial Behavior: Conduct Disorder, Delinquency, and Violence in the Dunedin Longitudinal Study.* Cambridge, England: Cambridge University Press.
National Research Council
  1996   *Understanding Violence Against Women,* N.A. Crowell and A.W. Burgess, eds. Panel on Research on Violence Against Women, Committee on Law and Justice, Commission on Behavioral and Social Sciences and Education. Washington, DC: National Academy Press.
Petrie, C., and J. Garner
  1990   Is violence preventable? Pp. 164-184 in *Family Violence: Research and Public Policy Issues,* D.J. Besharov, ed. Washington, DC: The American Enterprise Institute.
Rennison, C.M.
  2003   *Intimate Partner Violence, 1993-2001.* Crime Data Brief. Washington, DC: Bureau of Justice Statistics, U.S. Department of Justice.
  2001   *Criminal Victimization 2000: Changes 1999-2000 with Trends 1993-2000.* Washington, DC: Bureau of Justice Statistics, U.S. Department of Justice.
Tjaden, P., and N. Thoennes
  2000   *Extent, Nature, and Consequences of Intimate Partner Violence: Findings from the National Violence Against Women Survey.* Washington, DC: U.S. Department of Justice, National Institute of Justice. Available online at http://www.ncjrs.org/pdffiles1/nij/181867.pdf.

CHAPTER 2

Annest, J.L., and J.A. Mercy
  1998   Use of national data systems for firearm-related injury surveillance. *American Journal of Preventive Medicine* 15(3S):17-30.
Bachman, R.
  2000   A comparison of annual incidence rates and contextual characteristics of intimate-partner violence against women from the National Crime Victimization Survey (NCVS) and the National Violence Against Women Survey (NVAWS). *Violence Against Women* 6:815-838.
Bachman, R., and B. Taylor
  1994   The measurement of family violence and rape by the redesigned National Crime Victimization Survey. *Justice Quarterly* 11:701-714.
Browne, A., A. Salomon, and S.S. Bassuk
  1999   The impact of recent partner violence on poor women's capacity to maintain work. *Violence Against Women* 5:393-426.
Bureau of Justice Statistics
  2002   *Homicide Trends in the U.S.: Additional Information About the Data.* Available online at http://www.ojp.usdoj.gov/bjs/homicide/addinfo.htm.
  2000   *Criminal Victimization in the United States, 1993-1999.* Washington, DC: Office of Justice Programs, U.S. Department of Justice.
Campbell, J.
  2002   *Identifying Risk Factors for Femicide in Violent Intimate Relationships: Preliminary Data.* Baltimore, MD: Johns Hopkins University School of Nursing. Available online at http://www.son.jhmi.edu/research/CNR/Homicide/main.htm.
Campbell, J.C., S. Martin, B. Moracco, and J. Maganello
  2002a *Violence Against Women Data Sets That Allow Examination of Life Stage Patterns of Intimate Partner Violence Victimization.* Paper prepared for the Workshop on Issues in Research on Violence Against Women, The National Academies, Washington, DC, January 3-4.

Campbell, J., A. Snow Jones, J. Dienemann, J. Kub, J. Schollenberger, P. O'Campo, A. Carlson Gielen, and C. Wynne
2002b Intimate partner violence and physical health consequences. *Archives of Internal Medicine* 162:1157-1163.

Coker, A.L., P.H. Smith, R.E. McKeown, and M.J. King
2000 Frequency and correlates of intimate partner violence by type: Physical, sexual and psychological battering. *American Journal of Public Health* 90:553-559.

Cook, S.L.
2000 *Investigating the Roles of Context and Meaning in Violence Against Women.* Paper prepared for the Gender Symmetry Workshop, National Institute of Justice, Washington, DC, November 20.

Danielson, K.K., T.E. Moffitt, A. Caspi, and P.A. Silva
1998 Comorbidity between abuse of an adult and DSM-III-R mental disorders: Evidence from an epidemiological study. *American Journal of Psychiatry* 155:131-133.

Dawson, M.
2002 *Femicide: The Lethal Victimization of Women.* Paper prepared for the Workshop on Issues in Research on Violence Against Women, The National Academies, Washington, DC, January 3-4.

Diaz-Olavarrieta, C., J.C. Campbell, C. Garcia de la Cadena, F. Paz, and A. Villa
1999 Domestic violence against patients with chronic neurologic disorders. *Archives of Neurology* 56:681-685.

Dugan, L., and R. Apel
2002 *An Exploratory Study of the Violent Victimization of Women: Race/Ethnicity, Situational Context, and Injury.* Paper prepared for the Workshop on Issues in Research on Violence Against Women, The National Academies, Washington, DC, January 3-4.

Dugan, L., D. Nagin, and R. Rosenfeld
1999 Explaining the decline in intimate partner homicide: The effects of changing domesticity, women's status, and domestic violence resources. *Homicide Studies* 3:187-214.
2000 *Exposure Reduction or Backlash? The Effects of Domestic Violence Resources on Intimate Partner Homicide.* (A Report to the National Institute of Justice.) Washington, DC: U.S. Department of Justice.

Eby, K.K.
1996 *Experiences of Abuse and Stress: A Path Model of their Joint Effects on Women's Psychological and Physical Health.* Unpublished doctoral dissertation, Michigan State University.

Elliott, D.S., D. Huizinga, and B. Morse
1986 Self-reported violent offending: A descriptive analysis of juvenile violent offenders and their offending careers. *Journal of Interpersonal Violence* 1:472-514.

Felson, R.B., and S.F. Messner
1996 To kill or not to kill? Lethal outcomes in injurious attacks. *Criminology* 34:519-545.

Fisher, B.S., F.T. Cullen, and M.G. Turner
2000 *The Sexual Victimization of College Women.* Washington, DC: National Institute of Justice and Bureau of Justice Statistics, U.S. Department of Justice.

Gelles, R.J.
1987 *Family Violence,* 2nd ed. Thousand Oaks, CA: Sage.

Gelles, R.J., and M.A. Straus
1988 *Intimate Violence.* New York: Touchstone Books.

Golding, J.M.
1996 Sexual assault history and women's reproductive and sexual health. *Psychological Women Quarterly* 20:101-121.

1999 Intimate partner violence as a risk factor for mental disorders: A meta-analysis. *Journal of Family Violence* 14:99-132.

Greenfeld, L.A., M.R. Rand, D. Craven, P. Klaus, C. Perkins, C. Ringel, G. Warchol, and C. Maston
   1998 *Violence by Intimates: Analysis of Data on Crimes by Current or Former Spouses, Boyfriends, and Girlfriends.* Washington, DC: U.S. Department of Justice.

Hathaway, J.E., L.A. Mucci, J.G. Silverman, D.R. Brooks, R. Mathews, and C.A. Pavlos
   2000 Health status and health care use of Massachusetts women reporting partner abuse. *American Journal of Preventive Medicine* 19:302-307.

Infante, D., T.A. Chandler, and J.E. Rudd
   1989 Test of an argumentative skill deficiency model of interpersonal violence. *Communication Monograph* 56:163-177.

Jacobson, N., and J. Gottman
   1998 *When Men Batter Women: New Insights into Ending Abusive Relationships.* New York: Simon and Schuster.

Johnson, M.P.
   1995 Patriarchal terrorism and common couple violence: Two forms of violence against women. *Journal of Marriage and the Family* 57:283-294.

Kleck, G., and K. McElrath
   1991 The effects of weaponry on human violence. *Social Forces* 69:669-692.

Koss, M.P., and L. Heslet
   1992 Somatic consequences of violence against women. *Archives of Family Medicine* 1:53-59.

Kruttschnitt, C.
   2002 Women's involvement in serious interpersonal violence. *Aggression and Violent Behavior* 7:529-565.

Lemon, S.C., W. Verhoek-Oftedahl, and E.F. Donnelly
   2002 Preventive healthcare use, smoking, and alcohol use among Rhode Island women experiencing intimate partner violence. *Journal of Women's Health and Gender-Based Medicine* 11(6):555-562.

Letourneau, E.J., M. Holmes, and J. Chasedunn-Roark
   1999 Gynecologic health consequences to victims of interpersonal violence. *Women's Health Issues* 9:115-120.

Lloyd, S.A., and B.C. Emery
   2000 *The Dark Side of Courtship: Physical and Sexual Aggression.* Thousand Oaks, CA: Sage.

Menard, S.
   2002 Short- and long-term consequences of adolescent victimization. In *Youth Violence Research Bulletin.* Washington, DC: Office of Juvenile Justice and Delinquency Prevention and Centers for Disease Control and Prevention.

Moffitt, T.E., and A. Caspi
   1999 *Findings About Partner Violence from the Dunedin Multidisciplinary Health and Development Study.* Research In Brief. Washington, DC: National Institute of Justice, U.S. Department of Justice.

National Research Council
   1996 *Understanding Violence Against Women,* N.A. Crowell and A.W. Burgess, eds. Panel on Research on Violence Against Women, Committee on Law and Justice, Commission on Behavioral and Social Sciences and Education. Washington, DC: National Academy Press.

Plichta, S.B., and C. Abraham
   1996 Violence and gynecologic health in women <50 years old. *American Journal of Obstetrics and Gynecology* 174:903-907.

Rand, M.R.
  1997   *Violence-Related Injuries Treated in hospital Emergency Departments.* Bureau of Justice Statistics Special Report. Washington, DC: U.S. Department of Justice.
Rennison, C.M.
  2001   *Violent Victimization and Race, 1993.* BJS Special Report. Washington, DC: Bureau of Justice Statistics, U.S. Department of Justice.
  2002   *Criminal Victimization 2001: Changes 2000-01 with Trends 1993-2001.* Washington, DC: Bureau of Justice Statistics, U.S. Department of Justice.
  2003   *Intimate Partner Violence, 1993-2001.* Crime Data Brief. Washington, DC: Bureau of Justice Statistics, U.S. Department of Justice.
Rennison, C.M., and S. Welchans
  2000   *Intimate Partner Violence.* BJS Special Report. Washington, DC: Bureau of Justice Statistics, U.S. Department of Justice.
Richie, B.E.
  1996   *Compelled to Crime: The Gender Entrapment of Battered Black Women.* New York: Routledge.
Smith, P.H., J.B. Smith, and J.L. Earp
  1999   Beyond the measurement trap: A reconstructed conceptualization and measurement of woman battering. *Psychology of Women Quarterly* 23:177-193.
Statistics Canada
  1993   *Violence Against Women Survey.* Available online at http://stcwww.statcan.ca/english/sdds/3896.htm.
Straus, M.A.
  1979   Measuring intrafamily conflict and violence: The Conflict Tactics Scales. *Journal of Marriage and the Family* 41:75-88.
Straus, M.A., and R.J. Gelles
  1986   Societal change and change in family violence from 1975 to 1985 as revealed by two national surveys. *Journal of Marriage and the Family* 48:465-479.
  1992   *Physical Violence in American Families: Risk Factors and Adaptations to Violence.* New Brunswick, NJ: Transaction Publishers.
Straus, M.A., R.J. Gelles, and S.K. Steinmetz
  1988   *Behind Closed Doors: Violence in the American Family.* Thousand Oaks, CA: Sage.
Sullivan, C.M., C. Tan, J. Basta, M. Rumptz, and W.S. Davidson II
  1992   An advocacy intervention program for women with abusive partners: Initial evaluation. *American Journal of Community Psychology* 20:309-332.
Sutherland, C.A., C.M. Sullivan, and D.K. Bybee
  2001   Effects of intimate partner violence versus poverty on women's health. *Violence Against Women* 7:1122-1143.
Sutherland, C., D. Bybee, and C. Sullivan
  1998   The long-term effects of battering on women's health. *Womens Health* 4:41-70.
Tedeschi, J.T., and R.B. Felson
  1994   *Violence, Aggression, and Coercive Actions.* Washington, DC: American Psychological Association.
Tjaden, P., and N. Thoennes
  1998   *Prevalence, Incidence, and Consequences of Violence Against Women: Findings from the National Violence Against Women Survey.* Research in Brief. Washington, DC: National Institute of Justice.
  1999   *Violence and Threats of Violence Against Women and Men in the United States, 1994-1996: Machine-Readable Codebook.* Ann Arbor, MI: National Institute of Justice and the Inter-University Consortium for Political and Social Research.

2000   *Full Report of the Prevalence, Incidence, and Consequences of Violence Against Women.* Report from the National Institute of Justice and the Centers for Disease Control and Prevention. Washington, DC: U.S. Department of Justice.
Wilkinson, D., and S. Hamerschlag
2002   *Situational Determinants in Intimate Violence.* Paper presented at the Workshop on Issues in Research on Violence Against Women, National Research Council, Washington, DC, January 3-4.
Wilkinson, D.L., and J. Fagan
2001   A theory of violent events. Pp. 169-197 in *The Process and Structure of Crime*, R. Meier and L. Kennedy, eds. New Brunswick, NJ: Transaction Publishers.

CHAPTER 3

Baskin, D., and I. Sommers
1998   *Casualties of Community Disorder.* Boulder, CO: Westview Press.
Benson, M.L., G.L. Fox, A. DeMaris, and J. Van Wyk
2003   Neighborhood disadvantage, individual economic distress, and violence against women in intimate relationships. *Journal of Quantitative Criminology* 19(3):207-235.
Block, C.R., and A. Christakos
1995   Intimate partner homicide in Chicago over 29 years. *Crime and Delinquency* 41(4):496-526.
Browne, A., and K.R. Williams
1989   Exploring the effect of resource availability and the likelihood of female-perpetrated homicides. *Law & Society Review* 23:75-118.
Browning, C.R.
In   The span of collective efficacy: Extending social disorganization theory to partner
press   violence. *Journal of Marriage and the Family*.
Costanzo, M., W. Halperin, and N. Gale
1986   Criminal mobility and the directional component in journeys to crime. In *Metropolitan Crime Patterns*, R. Figlio, S. Hakim, and G. Rengert, eds. Monsey, NY: Criminal Justice Press.
Coulton, C., and S. Padney
1992   Geographic concentration of poverty and risk to children in urban neighborhoods. *American Behavioral Scientist* 35:238-257.
Coulton, C., J. Korbin, M. Su, and J. Chow
1995   Community level factors and child maltreatment. *Child Development* 66:1262-1276.
Dekeseredy, W., M.D. Schwartz, S. Alvi, and E.A. Tomaszewski
2003   Perceived collective efficacy in public housing. *Criminal Justice* 3:5-27.
Dugan, L., D. Nagin, and R. Rosenfeld
2000   Explaining the decline in intimate partner homicide: The effects of changing domesticity, women's status, and domestic violence resources. *Homicide Studies* 3(3):187-214.
Fagan, J.
1993   Social structure and spouse assault. Pp. 209-254 in *The Socio-economics of Crime and Justice*, B. Forst, ed. New York: M.A. Sharpe.
Fagan, J., J. Medina, and S. Wilt
2002   *The Social Ecology of Lethal and Non-lethal Violence Against Women in NYC (1990-1997).* Final report to the National Institute of Justice. Washington, DC: National Institute of Justice.

Garbarino, J., and D. Sherman
  1980   High-risk neighborhoods and high-risk families: The human ecology of child maltreatment. *Child Development* 51:188-198.
Kocsis, R., and H. Irwin
  1997   An analysis of spatial patterns in serial rape, arson, and burglary. *Psychiatry, Psychology, and Law* 4(2):195-206.
LeBeau, J.L.
  1979   *The Spatial Dynamics of Rape: The San Diego Example.* Ann Arbor, MI: Michigan State University.
  1985   Some problems with measuring and describing rape presented by the serial offender. *Justice Quarterly* 2(3):385-398.
  1987   Patterns of stranger and serial rape offending: Factors distinguishing apprehended and at-large offenders. *Journal of Criminal Law and Criminology* 78(2):309-326.
  1992   Case studies illustrating spatial-temporal analysis of serial rapists. *Police Studies* 15(3):124-145.
Macmillan, R., and R. Gartner
  1999   When she brings home the bacon: Labor-force participation and the risk of spousal violence against women. *Journal of Marriage and the Family* 61:947-958.
Massey, D., and N. Denton
  1993   *American Apartheid. Segregation and the Making of the Underclass.* Cambridge, MA: Harvard University Press.
Maxwell, C.D., J.H. Garner, and J.A. Fagan
  2001   *The Effects of Arrest on Intimate Partner Violence: New Evidence from the Spouse Assault Replication Program.* Research in Brief. Washington, DC: U.S. Department of Justice, Office of Justice Programs,.
Mears, D.P., M.J. Carlson, G.W. Holden, and S.D. Harris
  2001   The effects of individual and contextual factors and type of legal intervention. *Journal of Interpersonal Violence* 16:1260-1283.
Medina, J.
  2002a *Social and Ecological Risks of Domestic and Non-domestic Violence Against Women in New York City.* Doctoral dissertation, School of Criminal Justice, Rutgers University.
  2002b *The Social Geography of Violence Against Women.* Paper prepared for the Workshop on Issues in Research on Violence Against Women, The National Academies, Washington, DC, January 3-4.
Miles-Doan, R.
  1998   Violence between spouses and intimates: Does neighborhood context matter? *Social Forces* 77(2):623-645.
Mowrer, E.R.
  1927   *Family Disorganization. An Introduction to the Sociological Analysis.* Chicago: Chicago University Press.
Myers, W.C., A.W. Burgess, and J.A. Nelson
  1998   Criminal and behavioral aspects of juvenile sexual homicide. *Journal of Forensic Sciences* 43(2):340-347.
Rand, A.
  1984   *Patterns in Juvenile Delinquency: A Spatial Perspective.* Washington, DC: U.S. Department of Justice.
Rennison, C.M, and S. Welchans
  2000   *Intimate Partner Violence.* BJS Special Report. Washington, DC: Bureau of Justice Statistics, U.S. Department of Justice.

Rossmo, K.
  1995   Place, space, and police investigations: Hunting serial violent criminals. In *Crime and Place*, J. Eck and D. Weisburd, eds. Monsey, NY: Criminal Justice Press.
Sampson, R.J., and D. Jeglum Bartusch
  1998   Legal cynicism and (subcultural?) tolerance of deviance: The neighborhood context of racial differences. *Law and Society Review* 32:777-804.
Sampson, R.J., S. Raudenbush, and F. Earls
  1997   Neighborhoods and violent crime: A multilevel study of collective efficacy. *Science* 277:918-924.
Sherman, L.W., and D.A. Smith
  1992   Legal and informal control of domestic violence. *American Sociological Review* 57:680-690.
Simcha-Fagan, O., and J.E. Schwartz
  1986   Neighborhood and delinquency: An assessment of contextual effects. *Criminology* 24(4):667-703.
Stets, J.E.
  1991   Cohabiting and marital aggression: The role of social isolation. *Journal of Marriage and the Family* 53:669-680.
Stokes, R., and A. Chevan
  1996   Female-headed families: Social and economic context of racial differences. *Journal of Urban Affairs* 18(3):245-268.
Straus, M.A., R. Gelles, and S. Steinmetz
  1980   *Behind Closed Doors: Violence in the American Family*. Garden City, NY: Anchor Press, Doubleday.
Sullivan, M.
  1989   Absent fathers in the inner city. *Annals of the American Academy of Political and Social Science* 501:48-58.
  1993   Culture and class as determinants of out-of-wedlock childbearing and poverty during late adolescence. *Journal of Research on Adolescence* 3(3):295-316.
Taylor, R.B., and J. Covington
  1988   Neighborhood changes in ecology and violence. *Criminology* 26(4):553-589.
Thompson, M.P., N.J. Kaslow, J.B. Kingree, A. Rashid, R. Puett, D. Jacobs, and A. Matthews
  2000   Partner violence, social support, and distress among inner-city African American women. *American Journal of Community Psychology* 28(1):127-143.
Tjaden, P., and N. Thoennes
  2000   *Extent, Nature, and Consequences of Intimate Partner Violence. Findings from the National Violence Against Women Survey*. Washington, DC: U.S. Department of Justice, National Institute of Justice.
Tucker, M.B., and C. Mitchell-Kernan, eds.
  1995   *The Decline in Marriage Among African-Americans*. New York: Russell Sage Foundation.
Warren, J., R. Reboussin, R. Hazelwood, A. Cummings, N. Gibbs, and S. Trumbetta
  1998   Crime scene and distance correlates of serial rape. *Journal of Quantitative Criminology* 14(1):35-59.
Williams, K.R., and R. Hawkins
  1989a   The meaning of arrest for wife assault. *Criminology* 27:163-181.
  1989b   Controlling male aggression in intimate relationships. *Law & Society Review* 23:591-612.
  1992   Wife assault: Costs of arrest and the deterrence process. *Journal of Research in Crime and Delinquency* 29:292-310.

Wooldredge, J., and A. Thistlethwaite
  2002 Reconsidering domestic violence recidivism: Conditioned effects of legal controls by individual and aggregate levels of stake in conformity. *Journal of Quantitative Criminology* 18:46-70.

Zuravin, S.J.
  1989 The ecology of child abuse and neglect: Review of the literature and presentation of data. *Violence and Victims* 4:101-120.

CHAPTER 4

Bachman, R., R. Paternoster, and S. Ward
  1992 The rationality of sexual offending: Testing a deterrence/rational choice conception of sexual assault. *Law and Society Review* 26:343-372.

Baron, L., and M.A. Straus
  1989 *Four Theories of Rape in American Society.* New Haven, CT: Yale University Press.

Berk, R.A., A. Campbell, R. Klap, and B. Western
  1992 The deterrent effects of arrest in incidents of domestic violence: A Bayesian analysis of four field experiments. *American Sociological Review* 57:698-708.

Blair, A.K.
  1996 No: Grandstanding does not offer a solution. (Domestic violence: Should victims be forced to testify against their will?) *ABA Journal* 82:46.

Block, R.
  2002 *Data to Support New Prevention and Intervention Strategies.* Paper prepared for the Workshop on Advancing Research on Violence Against Women, The National Academies, Washington, DC, January 3-4.

Bloom, M.
  1981 *Primary Prevention: The Possible Science.* Englewood Cliffs, NJ: Prentice-Hall.

Bonnie, R.J.
  1981 The meaning of decriminalization: A review of the law. *Contemporary Drug Problems* 10:277-299.

Bowman, C.G.
  1992 The arrest experiments: A feminist critique. *Journal of Criminal Law and Criminology* 83:201-208.

Braga, A.A., D.M. Kennedy, E.J. Waring, and A.M. Piehl
  2001 Problem-oriented policing, deterrence, and youth violence: An evaluation of Boston's Operation Ceasefire. *Journal of Research in Crime and Delinquency* 38(3):195-225.

Breitenbecher, K.H.
  2000 Sexual assault on college campuses: Is an ounce of prevention enough. *Applied & Preventive Psychology* 9(1):23-52.

Bureau of Justice Statistics
  2002 *Homicide Trends in the U.S.* Available online at http://www.ojp.usdoj.gov/bjs/homicide/intimates.htm#intprop.

Campbell, J.
  1992 Wife battering: Cultural contexts verses Western social sciences. In *Sanctions and Sanctuary: Cultural Perspectives on the Beating of Wives*, C. Ayers, J.K. Brown, and J. Campbell, eds. Boulder, CO: Westview Press.

Carmody, D.C., and K.R. Williams
  1988 Wife assault and perception of sanctions. *Violence and Victims* 2:25-38.

Chaney, C.K., and G.H. Saltzstein
  1998   Democratic control and bureaucratic responsiveness: The police and domestic vio-
          lence. *American Journal of Political Science* 42:745.
Connolly, C., S. Huzurbazar, and T. Routh-McGee
  2000   Multiple parties in domestic violence situations and arrest. *Journal of Criminal Jus-
          tice* 28:181.
Cook, P.J.
  1980   Research in criminal deterrence: Laying the groundwork for the second decade. In
          Crime and Justice: An Annual Review of Research, vol. 2, N. Morris and M. Tonry,
          eds. Chicago: University of Chicago Press.
Cretney, A., and G. Davis
  1997   The significance of compellability in the prosecution of domestic assault. *British
          Journal of Criminology* 37:75.
Dugan, L., and R. Apel
  2002   *An Exploratory Study of the Violent Victimization of Women: Race/Ethnicity, Situ-
          ational Context, and Injury.* Paper prepared for the Workshop on Issues in Re-
          search on Violence Against Women, The National Academies, Washington, DC,
          January 3-4.
Dunford, F.W., W.D. Huizinga, and D.S. Elliott
  1990   The role of arrest in domestic assault: The Omaha experiment. *Criminology* 28:183-
          206.
Eck, J.E., and D. Weisburd
  1995   Crime places in crime theory. Pp. 1-33 in *Crime and Place*, J.E. Eck and D. Weisburd,
          eds. Monsey, NY: Criminal Justice Press.
Ellis, A.L., C.S. O'Sullivan, and B.A. Sowards
  1992   The impact of contemplated exposure to survivor of rape on attitudes towards
          rape. *Journal of Applied Social Psychology* 22:889-895.
Fagan, J.A.
  1989   Cessation of family violence: Deterrence and dissuasion. Pp. 377-425 in *Family
          Violence*, L. Ohlin and M. Tonry, eds. Chicago: University of Chicago Press.
  1996   *The Criminalization of Domestic Violence: Promises and Limits.* Presented at the Con-
          ference on Criminal Justice Research and Evaluation. Washington, DC: National
          Institute of Justice.
Feder, L.
  1998   Police handling of domestic and nondomestic assault calls: Is there a case for dis-
          crimination? *Crime and Delinquency* 44:335.
Felson, M.
  1987   Routine activities and crime prevention in the developing metropolis. *Criminology*
          25(4):911-931.
Fonow, M.M., L. Richardson, and V.A. Wemmerus
  1992   Feminist rape education: Does it work? *Gender and Society* 6:108-121.
Ford, D.A.
  1991   Prosecution as a victim power resource: A note on empowering women in violent
          conjugal relationships. *Law and Society Review* 25:313.
Ford, D.A., and M.J. Regoli
  1992   The preventive impacts of policies for prosecuting wife batterers. Pp. 181-208 in
          Domestic Violence: The Changing Criminal Justice Response, E.S. Buzawa and C.G.
          Buzawa, eds. Westport, CT: Auburn House.
Frisch, L.A.
  1992   Research that succeeds, policies that fail. *Journal of Criminal Law and Criminology*
          83:209-216.

Garner, J.H., and C.D. Maxwell
  2000   What are the lessons of the police arrest studies? *Journal of Aggression, Maltreatment & Trauma* 4:83-114.
Garner, J.H., J.A. Fagan, and C.C. Maxwell
  1995   Published findings from the Spouse Assault Replication Program: A critical review. *Journal of Quantitative Criminology* 11:3-28.
Garofalo, J.
  1987   Reassessing the lifestyle model of criminal victimization. Pp. 23-43 in *Positive Criminology*, M.R. Gottfredson and T. Hirschi, eds. Thousand Oaks, CA: Sage.
Goldberg, C.
  2001   In some states, sex offenders serve more than their time. *The New York Times on the Web*, 14th April. Available online at http://www.nytimes.com/2001/04/22/national/212mole.html.
Goodman, L., L. Bennett, and M.A. Dutton
  1999   Obstacles to victims' cooperation with the criminal prosecution of their abusers: The role of social support. *Violence and Victims* 14:427.
Gosselin, D.K.
  2000   *Heavy Hands: An Introduction to the Crimes of Domestic Violence.* Upper Saddle River, NJ: Prentice Hall.
Grasmick, H.G., and G.J. Bryjak
  1980   The deterrent effect of perceived severity of punishment. *Social Forces* 59:471-491.
Grasmick, H.G., R.J. Bursik, Jr., and K.A. Kinsey
  1991   Shame and embarrassment as deterrents to noncompliance with the law. *Environment and Behavior* 23:223-251.
Hanna, C.
  1996   No right to choose: Mandated victim participation in domestic violence prosecutions. *Harvard Law Review* 109:1849.
Hirschel, J.D., and I.W. Hutchison, III
  2001   The relative effects of offense, offender, and victim variables on the decision to prosecute domestic violence cases. *Violence Against Women* 7:46.
Hirschel, J.D., I.W. Hutchison III, C.W. Dean, J.J. Kelley, and C.E. Pesackis
  1991   *Charlotte Spouse Assault Replication Project* (Final Report, Grant No. 87-IJ-CK-K004). Washington, DC: National Institute of Justice.
Institute of Medicine
  1999   *Reducing the Burden of Injury: Advancing Prevention and Treatment.* R. Bonnie, C. Fulco, and C. Liverman, eds. Washington, DC: National Academy Press.
Kane, R.J.
  1999   Patterns of arrest in domestic violence encounters: Identifying a police decision-making model. *Journal of Criminal Justice* 27:65.
Kayitsinga, J., and C.D. Maxwell
  2000   *Sexual Assault Surveillance System* (Violence and Intentional Injury Prevention Programs No. 3(1)). East Lansing, MI: Michigan State University.
Kennedy, D.M., A.A. Braga, and A.M. Piehl
  2001   Developing and implementing Operation Ceasefire. In *Reducing Gun Violence: The Boston Gun Project's Operation Ceasefire*. Washington, DC: National Institute of Justice, U.S. Department of Justice.
Lackey, C., and K.R. Williams
  1995   Social bonding and the cessation of partner violence across generations. *Journal of Marriage and the Family* 57:295-305.
LeBeau, J.L.
  1994   The oscillation of police calls to domestic disputes with time and the temperature humidity index. *Journal of Crime and Justice* 17(1):1-13.

Lemon, N.K.D., ed.
    1996   *Domestic Violence Law: A Comprehensive Overview of Cases and Sources.* San Francisco: Austin & Winfield.

Lerman, L.G.
    1992   The decontextualization of domestic violence. *Journal of Criminal Law and Criminology* 83:217-240.

Lieb, R., and S. Matson
    1998   *Sexual Predators Commitment Laws in the United States: 1998 Update* (Tech. Rep. No. 98-09-1101). Olympia, WA: Washington State Institute for Public Policy.

Loh, W.D.
    1981   What has reform of rape legislation wrought?: A truth in criminal labeling. *Journal of Social Issues* 37(4):28-52.

Maxwell, C.D., and L.A. Post
    2002   *An Assessment of Efforts to Prevent Violence Against Women.* Paper prepared for the Workshop on Issues in Research on Violence Against Women, The National Academies, Washington, DC, January 3-4.

Maxwell, C.D., J.H. Garner, and J.A. Fagan
    2001   *The Effects of Arrest on Intimate Partner Violence: New Evidence from the Spouse Assault Replication Program.* Washington, DC: U.S. Department of Justice, Office of Justice Programs.

McCall, G.
    1993   Risk factors and sexual assault prevention. *Journal of Interpersonal Violence* 8:277-295.

Miethe, T.D.
    1994   *SUNY Series in Deviance and Social Control.* Albany, NY: State University of New York Press.

Mills, L.G.
    1998   Mandatory arrest and prosecution policies for domestic violence: A critical literature review and the case for more research to test victim empowerment approaches. *Criminal Justice and Behavior* 25:306.

Nagin, D.S.
    1998   Criminal deterrence research at the outset of the twenty-first century. Pp. 1-42 in *Crime and Justice: A Review of Research,* M. Tonry, ed. Chicago: University of Chicago Press.

Nagin, D.S., and R. Paternoster
    1993   Enduring individual differences and rational choice theories of crime. *Law and Society Review* 27:467-496.

National Institute of Justice
    1997   *Solicitation for Evaluation of Arrest Policies Program Under the Violence Against Women Act* (Solicitation). Washington, DC: U.S. Department of Justice, Office of Justice Programs, National Institute of Justice (8).

National Research Council
    1996   *Understanding Violence Against Women,* N.A. Crowell and A.W. Burgess, eds. Panel on Research on Violence Against Women, Committee on Law and Justice, Commission on Behavioral and Social Sciences and Education. Washington, DC: National Academy Press.

    2001   *Informing America's Policy on Illegal Drugs: What We Don't Know Keeps Hurting Us,* C.F. Manski, J.V. Pepper, and C.V. Petrie, eds. Committee on Data and Research for Policy on Illegal Drugs. Washington, DC: National Academy Press.

National Research Council and Institute of Medicine
    1998   *Violence in Families: Assessing Prevention and Treatment Programs,* R.A. Chalk and P.A. King, eds. Committee on the Assessment of Family Violence Intervention, Board on Children, Youth, and Families. Washington, DC: National Academy Press.
Pate, A.M., and E.E. Hamilton
    1992   Formal and informal deterrents to domestic violence: The Dade County spouse assault experiment. *American Sociological Review* 57:691-697.
Paternoster, R., L.E. Saltzman, T.G. Chiricos, and G.P. Waldo
    1982   Perceived risk and deterrence: Methodological artifacts in perceptual deterrence research. *Journal of Criminal Law and Criminology* 73:1238-1258.
Pleck, E.
    1989   Criminal approaches to family violence, 1640-1980. Pp. 19-57 in *Family Violence,* L. Ohlin and M. Tonry, eds. Chicago: University of Chicago Press.
    1987   *Domestic Tyranny: The Making of Social Policy.* New York: Oxford University Press.
Roark, M.L.
    1987   Preventing violence on college campuses. *Journal of Counseling and Development* 65:367-371.
Robbins, K.
    1999   No-drop prosecution of domestic violence: Just good policy, or equal protection mandate? *Stanford Law Review* 52:205.
Ross, H.L.
    1982   *Deterring the Drinking Driver: Legal Policy and Social Control.* Lexington, MA: Heath.
Rozee, P.D., and M.P. Koss
    2002   Rape: A century of resistance. *Psychology of Women Quarterly* 25.
Sanday, R.P.
    1981   The socio-cultural context of rape: A cross-cultural study. *Journal of Social Issues* 37(4):5-27.
Schewe, P., and W. O'Donohue
    1993   Rape prevention: Methodological problems and new directions. *Clinical Psychology Review* 13:667-682.
Schmidt, J.D., and L.W. Sherman
    1993   Does arrest deter domestic violence. *American Behavioral Scientist* 36:601-609.
Schram, D.D., and C.D. Milloy
    1995   *Community Notification: A Study of Offender Characteristics and Recidivism.* Prepared for the Washington State Institute for Public Policy. Seattle, WA: Urban Policy Research.
Shenkel, W.M.
    1989   The rape crisis in apartment management. *Journal of Property Management* 54(3):44-48.
Sherman, L.W.
    1990   Police crackdowns: Initial and residual deterrence. In *Crime and Justice: A Review of the Research,* vol. 12, M. Tonry and N. Morris, eds. Chicago: University of Chicago Press.
    1992a   The influence or criminology on criminal law: Evaluating arrests for misdemeanor domestic violence. *Journal of Criminal Law and Criminology* 83:1-45.
    1992b   *Policing Domestic Violence: Experiments and Dilemmas.* New York: Free Press.
Sherman, L.W., and E.G. Cohen
    1989   The impact of research on legal policy: The Minneapolis Domestic Violence Experiments. *Law & Society Review* 23(1):117-144.

Sherman, L.W., D.A. Smith, J.D. Schmidt, and D.P. Rogan
    1992   Crime, punishment, and stake in conformity: Legal and informal control of do-
            mestic violence. *American Sociological Review* 57:680-690.
Thompson, M.E.
    1991   Self-defense against sexual coercion: Theory, research, and practice. Pp. 111-121 in
            Sexual Coercion: A Sourcebook on its Nature, Causes, and Prevention. Lanham, MD:
            Rowman and Littlefield.
Ullman, S.E.
    1997   Review and critique of empirical studies of rape avoidance. *Criminal Justice and
            Behavior* 24(2):177-204.
Williams, K.R.
    1992   Social sources of marital violence and deterrence: Testing an integrated theory of
            assaults between partners. *Journal of Marriage and the Family* 54:620-629.
Williams, K.R., and E. Conniff
    2002   *Legal Sanctions and the Violent Victimization of Women*. Paper prepared for the Work-
            shop on Issues in Research on Violence Against Women, The National Academies,
            Washington, DC, January 3-4.
Williams, K.R., and R. Hawkins
    1989a   Controlling male aggression in intimate relationships. *Law & Society Review* 23:591-
            612.
    1989b   The meaning of arrest for wife assault. *Criminology* 27:163-181.
    1992   Wife assault, costs of arrest, and the deterrence process. *Journal of Research in Crime
            and Delinquency* 292-310.
Woods, S., and D. Bower
    2001   College students' attitudes toward date rape and date rape backlash: Implications
            for prevention programs. *American Journal of Health Education* 32(4):194-198.
Zorza, J.
    1992   The criminal law of misdemeanor domestic violence. *Journal of Criminal Law and
            Criminology* 83(1):46-72.

CHAPTER 5

Babcock, J., C. Green, and C. Robie
    In   Does batterer's treatment work? A meta-analytic review of domestic violence out-
    press   come research. *Journal of Family Psychology* 13:46-59.
Barbaree, H.E., M.C. Seto, C.M. Langton, and E.J. Peacock
    2001   Evaluating the predictive accuracy of six risk assessment instruments for adult
            sex offenders. *Criminal Justice and Behavior* 28(4):490-521.
Brannen, S.J., and A. Rubin
    1996   Comparing the effectiveness of gender-specific and couples groups in a court-
            mandated spouse abuse treatment program. *Research on Social Work Practice*
            6(4):405-424.
Burton, D.L., and J. Smith-Darden
    2001   *North American Survey of Sexual Abuser Treatment and Models Summary Data*. Bran-
            don, VT: Safer Society Press.
Campbell, J.C.
    1986   Nursing assessment for risk of homicide with battered women. *Advances in Nurs-
            ing Science* 8(4):36-51.
    1995   Predicting homicide of and by battered women. In *Assessing Dangerousness: Vio-
            lence by Sexual Offenders, Batterers, and Child Abusers*, J.C. Campbell, ed. Thousand
            Oaks, CA: Sage.

Carrillo, R., and J. Tello
1998   *Family Violence and Men of Color*. New York: Springer.
Daly, J.E., and S. Pelowski
2000   Predictors of dropout among men who batter: A review of studies with implications for research and practice. *Violence and Victims* 15:137-160.
Davis, J.E., and B.G. Taylor
1999   Does batterer treatment reduce recidivism? A synthesis of the literature. *Women and Criminal Justice* 10:69-93.
Davis, R.C., B.G. Taylor, and C.D. Maxwell
2000   *Does Batterer Treatment Reduce Violence? A Randomized Experiment in Brooklyn*. Washington, DC: National Institute of Justice, U.S. Department of Justice.
de Becker, G.
1997   *The Gift of Fear: Survival Signals That Protect Us from Violence*. Boston, MA: Little, Brown & Co.
Dunford, F.W.
2000   The San Diego Navy Experiment: An assessment of interventions for men who assault their wives. *Journal of Consulting and Clinical Psychology* 68:468-476.
Dutton, D.G.
1995   Intimate abusiveness. *Clinical Psychology: Science and Practice* 2:207-224.
Dutton, D.G., and P.R. Kropp
2000   A review of domestic violence risk instruments. *Trauma Violence & Abuse* 1(2):171-181.
Edleson, J.L., and M. Syers
1990   Relative effectiveness of group treatments for men who batter. *Social Work Research and Abstracts* 26(2):10-17.
1991   The effects of group treatment for men who batter: An 18 month follow-up study. *Research on Social Work Practice* 1:227-243.
English, K., S. Pullen, and L. Jones, eds.
1996   *Managing Adult Sex Offenders: A Containment Approach*. Lexington, KY: American Probation and Parole Association.
Fagan, J.
1996   *The Criminalization of Domestic Violence: Promises and Limits*. Washington, DC: National Institute of Justice, U.S. Department of Justice.
Fedoroff, J.P., R. Wisner-Carlson, S. Dean, and S. Berlin
1992   Medroxy-progesterone acetate in the treatment of paraphilic sexual disorders: Rate of relapse in paraphilic men treated in long-term group psychotherapy with or without medroxy-progesterone acetate. *Journal of Offender Rehabilitation: Special Issue: Sex Offender Treatment: Psychological and Medical Approaches* 18(3-4):109-123.
Freeman-Longo R.E., S. Bird, W.F. Stevenson, and J.A. Fiske
1995   *1994 Nationwide Survey of Treatment Programs and Models*. Brandon, VT: Safer Society Press.
Gendreau, P., F.T. Cullen, and J. Bonta
1994   Intensive rehabilitation supervision: The next generation in community corrections? *Federal Probation* 58:72-78.
Gondolf, E.W.
1997   Batterer programs: What we know and need to know. *Journal of Interpersonal Violence* 12:83-98.
2001   Limitations of experimental evaluation of batterer programs. *Trauma, Violence, and Abuse* 2:79-88.
Gondolf, E.W., and R.J. White
2001   Batterer program participants who repeatedly reassault: Psychopathic tendencies and other disorders. *Journal of Interpersonal Violence* 16:361-380.

Hamberger, L.K., and J.E. Hastings
   1993   Court mandated treatment of men who assault their partners: Issues, controversies, and outcomes. In *Legal Response to Wife Assault*, N.Z. Hilton, ed. Thousand Oaks, CA: Sage.
Hanson, R.K., A. Gordon, A.J.R. Harris, J.K. Marques, W. Murphy, V.L. Quinsey, and M.C. Seto
   2000   *The 2000 ATSA Report on the Effectiveness of Treatment for Sexual Offenders.* Paper presented at the 19th Annual Research and Treatment Conference of the Association for the Treatment of Sexual Abusers, San Diego, CA, November 1-4.
Harlow, C.W.
   1999   Prior abuse reported by inmates and probationers. In *Bureau of Justice Statistics Selected Findings.* Washington, DC: U.S. Department of Justice.
Hart, B.
   1988   Beyond the "duty to warn": A therapist's "duty to protect" battered women and children. In *Feminist Perspectives on Wife Abuse*, K. Yllo and M. Bograd, eds. Thousand Oaks, CA: Sage.
Healey, K., C. Smith, and C. O'Sullivan
   1998   *Batterer Intervention: Program Approaches and Criminal Justice Strategies.* Washington, DC: National Institute of Justice.
Holtzworth-Munroe, A., and J.C. Meehan
   2002   *Typologies of Maritally Violent Men: A Summary of Current Knowledge and Suggestions for Future Research.* Paper prepared for the Workshop on Issues in Research on Violence Against Women, The National Academies, Washington, DC, January 3-4.
Holtzworth-Munroe, A., and G.L. Stuart
   1994   Typologies of male batterers: Three subtypes and the differences among them. *Psychological Bulletin* 116:476-497.
Holtzworth-Munroe, A., S.B. Beatty, and K. Anglin
   1995   The assessment and treatment of marital violence: An introduction for the marital therapist. Pp. 317-339 in *Clinical Handbook of Couple Therapy*, N.S. Jacobson and A.S. Gurman, eds. New York: Guilford.
Holtzworth-Munroe, A., J.C. Meehan, K. Herron, U. Rehman, and G.L. Stuart
   2000   Testing the Holtzworth-Munroe (1994) batterer typology. *Journal of Consulting and Clinical Psychology* 68:1000-1019.
Jones, A.S., and E.W. Gondolf
   In   Time-varying risk factors for re-assault among batterer program participants. *Journal of Family Violence.*
   press
Jones, R.L., C.M. Loredo, S.D. Johnson, and G.H. McFarlane-Nathan
   1999   A paradigm for culturally relevant sexual abuser treatment: An international perspective. Pp. 3-44 in *Cultural Diversity in Sexual Abuser Treatment: Issues and Approaches*, A.D. Lewis, ed. Brandon, VT: Safer Society Press.
Knight, R.A., and R.A. Prentky
   1990   Classifying sexual offenders: The development and corroboration of taxonomic models. Chapter 3 in *Handbook of Sexual Assault: Issues, Theories, and Treatment of the Offender*, W.L. Marshall, D.R. Laws, and H.E. Barbaree, eds. New York: Plenum Press.
Kropp, P.R., S.D. Hart, C.D. Webster, and D. Eaves
   1999   *Spousal Assault Risk Assessment Guide: User's Manual.* North Tonawanda, NY: Multi-Health Systems, Inc. and B.C. Institute Against Family Violence.
Kruttschnitt, C., and R. Gartner
   2003   Women's imprisonment. In *Crime and Justice: A Review of Research*, vol. 30, M. Tonry, ed. Chicago: University of Chicago Press.

Lattimore, P.K., C.A. Visher, and R.L. Linster
  1995   Predicting rearrest for violence among serious youthful offenders. *Journal of Research in Crime and Delinquency* 32:54-83.
Levesque, D.A.
  1998   *Violence Desistance Among Battering Men: Existing Interventions and the Application of the Transtheoretical Model of Change.* Doctoral dissertation, University of Rhode Island.
Lewis, A.D., ed.
  1999   *Cultural Diversity in Sexual Abuser Treatment: Issues and Approaches.* Brandon, VT: Safer Society Press.
Marques, J.K.
  1999   How to answer the question: "Does sex offender treatment work?" *Journal of Interpersonal Violence* 14(4):437-451.
Marshall, W.L.
  1999   Current status of North American assessment and treatment programs for sexual offenders. *Journal of Interpersonal Violence* 14:221-239.
Marshall, W.L, and G.A. Serran
  2000   Improving the effectiveness of sexual offender treatment. *Trauma, Violence, & Abuse* 1(3):203-222.
Marshall, W.L., Y.M. Fernandez, S.M. Hudson, and T. Ward
  1998   *Sourcebook of Treatment Programs for Sexual Offenders.* New York: Plenum Press.
McConaghy, N.
  1999   Methodological issues concerning evaluation of treatment for sexual offenders: Randomization, treatment dropouts, untreated controls, and within-treatment studies. *Sexual Abuse: Journal of Research & Treatment* 11(3):183-193.
McNeill, M.
  1987   Domestic violence: The skeleton in Tarasoff's closet. Pp. 197-217 in *Domestic Violence on Trial: Psychological and Legal Dimensions of Family Violence*, D.J. Sonkin, ed. New York: Springer.
Miller, R.D.
  1998   Forced administration of sex-drive reducing medications to sex offenders: Treatment or punishment. *Psychology, Public Policy, & Law: Special Issue: Sex Offenders: Scientific, Legal, and Policy Perspectives* 4(1-2):175-199.
Moffitt, T.E., and A. Caspi
  1998   Annotation: Implications of violence between intimate partners for child psychologists and psychiatrists. *Journal of Child Psychology and Psychiatry* 39(2):137-144.
Moffitt, T.E., A. Caspi, M. Rutter, and P.A. Silva
  2001   *Sex Differences in Antisocial Behavior: Conduct Disorder, Delinquency, and Violence in the Dunedin Longitudinal Study.* Cambridge, England: Cambridge University Press.
National Research Council
  1996   *Understanding Violence Against Women*, N.A. Crowell and A.W. Burgess, eds. Panel on Research on Violence Against Women, Committee on Law and Justice, Commission on Behavioral and Social Sciences and Education. Washington, DC: National Academy Press.
National Research Council and Institute of Medicine
  1998   *Violence in Families: Assessing Prevention and Treatment Programs*, R.A. Chalk and P.A. King, eds. Committee on the Assessment of Family Violence Intervention, Board on Children, Youth, and Families. Washington, DC: National Academy Press.
O'Leary, K.D., R.E. Heyman, and P.H. Neidig
  1999   Treatment of wife abuse: A comparison of gender-specific and conjoint approaches. *Behavior Therapy* 30:475-505.

Pirog-Good, M., and J. Stets-Kealey
  1985   Male batterers and battering prevention programs: A national survey. *Response to the Victimization of Women and Children* 8(3):8-12.
Prentky, R.A.
  1997   Arousal reduction in sexual offenders: A review of antiandrogen interventions. *Sexual Abuse: Journal of Research & Treatment* 9(4):335-347.
Risk and Needs Assessment
  1996   *Domestic Violence Inventory.* Phoenix, AZ: Risk and Needs Assessment, Inc.
Robinson, T., and F. Valcour
  1995   The use of depo-provera in the treatment of child molesters and sexually compulsive males. *Sexual Addiction & Compulsivity* 2(4):277-294.
Roehl, J., and K. Guertin
  2000   Intimate partner violence: The current use of risk assessments in sentencing offenders. *Justice System Journal* 21(2):171-198.
Rosenfeld, B.D.
  1992   Court-ordered treatment of spouse abuse. *Clinical Psychology Review* 12:205-226.
Saunders, D.G.
  1996   Feminist-cognitive-behavioral and process-psychodynamic treatments for men who batter: Interaction of abuser traits and treatment models. *Violence and Victims* 11:393-414.
Saunders, D.G., and J.C. Parker
  1989   Legal sanctions and treatment follow-through among men who batter: A multivariate analysis. *Social Work Research and Abstracts* 25(3):21-29.
Saunders, D.G., and R. Hamill
  2002   *Offender Interventions to End Violence Against Women: A Research Synthesis for Practitioners.* Paper prepared for the Workshop on Issues in Research on Violence Against Women, The National Academies, Washington, DC, January 3-4.
Stosny, S.
  1994   "Shadows of the heart": A dramatic video for the treatment resistance of spouse abuse. *Social Work* 39:686-694.
Taft, C.T., C.M. Murphy, J.D. Elliott, and M.C. Keaser
  2001   Race and demographic factors in treatment attendance for domestically abusive men. *Journal of Family Violence* 16:385-400.
Tolman, R.M., and G. Bhosley
  1991   The outcome of participation in a shelter-sponsored program for men who batter. In *Abused and Battered: Social and Legal Responses,* D. Knudsen and J. Miller, eds. New York: Aldine de Gruyter.
Tolman, R.M., and J.L. Edleson
  1995   Intervention for men who batter: A review of research. Pp. 262-274 in *Understanding Partner Violence,* S. Stith and M.A. Straus, eds. Minneapolis, MN: National Council on Family Relations.
Websdale, N.
  2000   *Lethality Assessment Tools: A Critical Analysis.* VAWnet, a project of the National Resource Center on Domestic Violence. Available online at http://www.vaw.umn.edu/Vawnet/lethality.htm.
Weisz, A.N., R.M. Tolman, and D.G. Saunders
  2000   Assessing the risk of severe domestic violence: The importance of survivors' predictions. *Journal of Interpersonal Violence* 15:75-90.
Williams, O.J.
  1994   Group work with African-American men who batter: Toward more ethnically sensitive practice. *Journal of Comparative Family Studies* 25:91-103.

Williams, O.J., and R.L. Becker
1994   Domestic partner abuse treatment programs and cultural competence: The results of a national survey. *Violence and Victims* 9:287-296.

CHAPTER 6

Moffitt, T.E., A. Caspi, M. Rutter, and P. Silva
2001   *Sex Differences in Antisocial Behavior: Conduct Disorder, Delinquency, and Violence in the Dunedin Longitudinal Study.* Cambridge, England: Cambridge University Press.
National Research Council
1996   *Understanding Violence Against Women,* N.A. Crowell and A.W. Burgess, eds. Panel on Research on Violence Against Women, Committee on Law and Justice, Commission on Behavioral and Social Sciences and Education. Washington, DC: National Academy Press.
Sampson, R.J., and D.J. Bartusch
1998   Legal cynicism and (subcultural?) tolerance of deviance: The neighborhood context of racial differences. *Law and Society Review* 32:777-804.
Shaw, C.R., and H.D. McKay
1942   *Juvenile Delinquency and Urban Areas.* Chicago: University of Chicago Press.

ADDENDUM

Archer, J.
2000   Sex differences in aggression between heterosexual partners: A meta-analytic review. *Psychological Bulletin* 126(5):651-680.
Brannen, S.J., and A. Rubin
1996   Comparing the effectiveness of gender-specific versus couples' groups in a court mandated spouse abuse treatment program. *Research on Social Work Practice* 6(4):405-424.
Dunford, F.W.
2000   The San Diego Navy experiment: An assessment of interventions for men who assault their wives. *Journal of Consulting and Clinical Psychology* 68(3):468-476.
Felson, R.B., and S.F. Messner
2000   The control motive in intimate partner violence. *Social Psychology Quarterly* 63(March):86-94.
Felson, R.B., S.F. Messner, and A. Hoskin
1999   The victim-offender relationship and calling the police in assaults. *Criminology* 37(4):931-948.
Finn, M.A., and L.J. Stalans
1997   The influence of gender and mental state on police decisions in domestic assault cases. *Criminal Justice and Behavior* 24(2):157.
Fyfe, J.F., D.A. Klinger, and J.M. Flavin
1997   Differential police treatment of male-on-female spousal violence. *Criminology* 35(3):455-473.
Healey, K., C. Smith, and C. O'Sullivan
1998   *Batterer Intervention: Program Approaches and Criminal Justice Strategies.* Washington, DC: National Institute of Justice, U.S. Department of Justice.
Klinger, D.A.
1995   Policing spousal assault. *Journal of Research in Crime and Delinquency* 32:308-324.

Lavoie, F., L. Vezina, C. Piche, and M. Boivin
   1995   Evaluation of a prevention program for violence in teen dating relationships. *Journal of Interpersonal Violence* 10:516-524.
Marvell, T.B., and C.E. Moody
   1999   Female and male homicide victimization rates: Comparing trends and regressors. *Criminology* 37(4):879-902.
McFarlane, J., K. Soeken, and W. Wiist
   2000   An evaluation of interventions to decrease intimate partner violence to pregnant women. *Public Health Nursing* 17:443-451.
Miller, N.
   1997   *Domestic Violence Legislation Affecting Police and Prosecutor Responsibilities in the United States: Inferences from a 50-State Review of State Statutory Codes.* Alexandria, VA: Institute for Law and Justice.
Mirrlees-Black, C.
   1999   *Domestic Violence: Findings from the British Crime Survey Self Completion Questionnaire.* London, England: Great Britain Home Office.
O'Leary, K.D.
   1999   Psychological abuse: A variable deserving critical attention in domestic violence. *Violence and Victims* 14:3-23.
Parker, B., J. McFarlane, K. Soeken, C. Silva, and S. Reel
   1999   Testing an intervention to prevent further abuse to pregnant women. *Research in Nursing and Health* 22:59-66.
Robinson, A.L., and M.S. Chandek
   2000   The domestic violence arrest decision: Examining demographic, attitudinal, and situational variables. *Crime and Delinquency* 46(1):18-37.
Shields, G., J. Baer, K. Leininger, J. Marlow, and P. DeKeyser
   1998   Interdisciplinary health care and female victims of domestic violence. *Social Work in Health Care* 27:27-48.
Sullivan, C.M., and D.I. Bybee
   1999   Reducing violence using community-based advocacy for women with abusive partners. *Journal of Consulting and Clinical Psychology* 67(1):43-53.
Wathen, C.N., and H.L. MacMillan
   2003   Interventions for violence against women: Scientific review. *Journal of the American Medical Association* 289:589-600.

APPENDIX
A

Biographical Sketches

Candace Kruttschnitt (*Chair*) is a professor in the Department of Sociology at the University of Minnesota. She has published widely on the subject of female offenders, including both reviews of research pertaining to gender differences in etiology and primary analyses of criminal court sanctions. Most recently, she has been finishing a study, with Professor Rosemary Gartner, of women's responses to imprisonment. Her current research interests focus on the law, criminology and deviance, and gender and life courses. She has published on topics that include gender and violence and the interaction between formal and informal social control. She has a B.A. in criminology from the University of California, Berkeley, and an M.S. and Ph.D. in sociology, both from Yale University.

Jeffrey A. Fagan is a professor of law and public health at Columbia University. For over two decades, his research and scholarship have focused on crime, law, and social policy. His current research examines error rates in capital punishment, racial profiling, and the jurisprudence of adolescent crime; community courts and therapeutic jurisprudence; and perceptions of the legitimacy of the criminal law. His past research has included studies of street gangs, drug selling, domestic violence, and the spatial analysis of adolescent violence. He is a member of the National Research Council's Committee on Law and Justice, the MacArthur Foundation's Research Network on Adolescent Development and Juvenile Justice, the Incarceration Working Group of the Russell Sage Foundation, and the National Consortium on Violence Research. From 1994 to 1998, he served on the Violence Study Section of the National Institute of Mental Health.

Mindy Thompson Fullilove is research psychiatrist at Columbia University, with a joint appointment as associate professor of Clinical Psychiatry and Public Health. She has been involved in research on substance abuse and HIV infection, including a study examining the access of minority women to AIDS resources, and on health risk due to lifetime trauma, violence, and environmental breakdown. She has completed a longitudinal study of housing resettlement in central Harlem involving the experiences of 10 families, as well as an interview study of over 100 men and women aimed at understanding their experiences of the violence epidemic in their neighborhood. Her current work includes an evaluation of the effectiveness of two interventions designed to improve environmental health, and a project aimed at delineating the process of spiritual awakening that occurs among participants in 12-step fellowship addiction treatment. She is a current member of the National Research Council's Board on Children, Youth, and Families.

Brenda L. McLaughlin is a research associate with the Committee on Law and Justice at the National Research Council. She has previously worked on projects on juvenile crime, school violence, policing, and improving data and research for drug policy. Ms. McLaughlin received a B.A. in sociology and Spanish from Juniata College in 1997, and an M.A. in sociology from American University in 1999.

Daniel S. Nagin is a professor of management at the H. J. Heinz III School of Public Policy and Management, Carnegie Mellon University, and the research director of the National Consortium on Violence Research. He has written widely on deterrence, developmental trajectories and criminal careers, tax compliance, and statistical methodology. He is a member of the National Research Council's Committee on Law and Justice and is also a coeditor of the widely cited report *Deterrence and Incapacitation: Estimating the Effect of Criminal Sanctions on Crime Rates* (1978). He is on the editorial board of five academic journals and a fellow of the American Society of Criminology. He has a B.S. in administrative and managerial sciences, an M.S. in industrial administration, and a Ph.D. in urban and public affairs from Carnegie Mellon University.

Carol V. Petrie, study director, serves as staff director of Committee on law and Justice, National Research Council (NRC), a position she has held since 1997. Prior to her work at the NRC, she was the director of Planning and Management at the National Institute of Justice (NIJ), responsible for policy development and administration. In 1994, she served as the Acting Director of NIJ during the transition between the Bush and Clinton Administrations. Throughout a 30-year career she has worked in the area of criminal justice research, statistics, and public policy, serving as a project officer and in administration at NIJ and at the Bureau of Justice Statistics. She has conducted research on violence, and managed numerous research projects on the development of criminal behavior, policy on illegal drugs, domestic violence, child abuse and neglect, transnational crime, and improving the operations of the criminal justice system.

APPENDIX
B

Workshop Agenda

Workshop on Advancing Research on Violence Against Women
The Committee on Law and Justice
and
The National Research Council's
Division of Behavioral and Social Sciences and Education

January 3–4, 2002

The Lecture Room
National Academy of Sciences
2101 Constitution Avenue NW
Washington, DC 20418

Thursday, January 3, 2002

8:30–9:15   **Welcome (pastries and coffee available)**

Jane Ross
Director
Center for Social and Economic Studies
National Research Council

Carol Petrie
Director
Committee on Law and Justice

Introduction—Objectives of Workshop

Candace Kruttschnitt
Workshop Chair
Department of Sociology
University of Minnesota

9:15–9:35 **VAWA'S Preventive Impacts: Research, Prospects, and Findings**

David Ford
Department of Sociology
Indiana University, Indianapolis

9:35–9:50 Comments

Adele Harrell
Director, Justice Policy Center
Urban Institute

9:50–10:20 Open Discussion

10:20–10:35 Break

10:35–10:55 **An Exploratory Study of the Violent Victimization of Women: Race/Ethnicity, Situational Context, and Injury**

Laura Dugan
Department of Criminology and Criminal Justice
University of Maryland

10:55–11:15 Comments

Ann Coker
School of Public Health
University of South Carolina

Colin Loftin
School of Criminal Justice
University at Albany

11:15–11:40 Open Discussion

11:40–12:00 **Life Course Violent Victimization—An Ethnographic Approach**

Patricia Munhall
Institute for Families in Society
University of South Carolina

12:00–12:15   **Violence Against and By Women**

              Beth Richie
              Department of Criminal Justice
              University of Illinois, Chicago

12:15–12:45   Open Discussion

12:45–2:15   Lunch

1:45–2:15   **Current Data Sets That Allow Examination of Life Stage
              Patterns of Intimate Partner Victimization**

              Jackie Campbell
              School of Nursing
              Johns Hopkins University

              Sandra Martin
              Department of Maternal and Child Health
              University of North Carolina

2:15–2:30   Comments

              Ross MacMillan
              Department of Sociology
              University of Minnesota

2:30–3:00   Open Discussion

3:00–3:15   Break

3:15–3:35   **The Social Geography of Violence Against Women**

              Juanjo Medina
              Criminology and Applied Social Science
              University of Manchester

3:35–3:50   Comments

              Michael Benson
              Division of Criminal Justice
              University of Cincinnati

3:50–4:20   Open Discussion

4:20–4:40   **Situational Determinants of Intimate Violence**

               Deanna Wilkinson
               Department of Criminal Justice
               Temple University

4:40–4:55   Comments

               Robert F. Meier
               Department of Criminal Justice
               University of Nebraska at Omaha

4:55–5:25   Open Discussion

5:25–5:30   **Wrap-Up**

               Candace Kruttschnitt

5:30   Adjourn

Friday, January 4, 2002

8:30–8:45   **Welcome (pastries and coffee available)**

8:45–9:05   **Legal Sanctions and the Violent Victimization of Women**

               Kirk R. Williams
               Robert Presley Center for Crime and Justice
               University of California, Riverside

9:05–9:20   Greg Pogarsky
               School of Criminal Justice
               University at Albany

9:20–9:50   Open Discussion

9:50–10:10   **An Assessment of Efforts to Prevent Violence Against Women**

                Christopher D. Maxwell
                School of Criminal Justice
                Michigan State University

10:10–10:30   Comments

                Alissa Worden
                School of Criminal Justice
                University at Albany

                John Firman
                Director of Research
                International Association of Chiefs of Police

10:30–10:55   Open Discussion

10:55–11:10   Break

11:10–11:30   **Community Epidemiology on Prevention**

                Ann Coker
                School of Public Health
                University of South Carolina

11:30–11:45   **Data to Support New Prevention and Intervention Strategies**

                Carolyn Rebecca Block
                Illinois Criminal Justice Information Authority

11:45–12:15   Open Discussion

12:15–12:35   **Motivations of Men Who Batter**

                Amy Holtzworth-Munroe
                Department of Psychology
                Indiana University–Bloomington

12:35–12:50   Comments

                Julie Horney
                School of Criminal Justice
                University of Nebraska at Omaha

12:50–1:50   **Working Lunch**
                Open Discussion

1:50–2:10   **Offender Interventions to End Violence Against Women:**
                A Research Synthesis for Practitioners

                Daniel G. Saunders
                School of Social Work
                University of Michigan

2:10–2:25   Comments

                Marty Friday
                Women's Center and Shelter
                Pittsburgh, PA

2:25–3:00   Open Discussion

3:00–3:15   Break

3:15– 3:35   **Femicide—The Murder of Women**

                Myrna Dawson
                Centre for Research on Violence and Conflict Resolution
                and Centre for Research on Violence Against Women
                and Children
                University of Western Ontario

3:35–3:50   Comments

                Bill McCarthy
                Department of Sociology
                University of California,Davis

3:50–4:10   Open Discussion

4:10–4:30   **Wrap-Up Discussion on Future Research Needs**

               Candace Kruttschnitt

4:30   Adjourn Public Meeting

Appendix
C

Commissioned Papers

Jacquelyn C. Campbell, Sandra Martin, Beth Moracco, and Jennifer Maganello. Violence Against Women Datasets That Allow Examination of Life Stage Patterns of Intimate Partner Violence Victimization.

Laura Dugan and Robert Apel. An Exploratory Study of the Violent Victimization of Women: Race/Ethnicity, Situational Context, and Injury.

Amy Holtzworth-Munroe and Jeffrey C. Meehan. Typologies of Maritally Violent Men: A Summary of Current Knowledge and Suggestions for Future Research.

Christopher D. Maxwell and Lori A. Post. An Assessment of Efforts to Prevent Violence Against Women.

Juanjo Medina. The Social Geography of Violence Against Women.

Daniel G. Saunders and Richard Hamill. Offender Interventions to End Violence Against Women: A Research Synthesis for Practitioners.

Deanna L. Wilkinson and Susan Hamerschlag. Situational Determinants in Intimate Violence.

Krik R. Williams and Elizabeth Conniff. Legal Sanctions and the Violent Victimization of Women.